DON'T BURN OUT BURN OUT STAND OUT

AN ENTREPRENEUR'S GUIDE TO SUCCESS WITHOUT SACRIFICE

BETHANY AINSLEY

R^ethink

First published in Great Britain in 2023
by Rethink Press (www.rethinkpress.com)

Cover image © Shutterstock | amasterphotographer

*Dedicated to my beautiful son Rory,
born during the writing of this book*

Contents

Introduction

Perhaps you always felt destined to be an entrepreneur, or maybe it was a calculated decision where you carefully weighed up the risks and rewards. Making those first steps can feel exciting and liberating, especially as you picture yourself pursuing your passion as a successful business owner. Perhaps you started your business for more flexibility, to be your own boss, to make more money or to help others.

To make their ambitions a reality, entrepreneurs are generally willing to work significantly more hours for themselves than they would if they were employees. Long hours, constant pressure to perform well and secure tangible results can take their toll on even the most resilient of business owners.

For busy, hardworking and ambitious entrepreneurs, finding balance is key to thriving in all areas of life, but it is also one of the biggest challenges. In today's society, it has become the norm to live a busy, fast-paced life. You may have found yourself working at an unsustainable pace, helping others more than you help yourself, burning the candle at both ends, or perhaps all of the above. This can be the catalyst for an easy journey towards burnout.

As a corporate wellbeing specialist and coach, many entrepreneurs come to me feeling overwhelmed, stressed or burned out. Others are looking for a better way to do business and achieve amazing results without the detriment of their health, wellbeing and personal lives.

Many business owners avoid taking time away from work to recharge because they fear that their business will suffer in their absence. If you can relate to this, it's important to remember that fatigue can lead to poor decision-making, low mood, irritability and illness, which can ultimately have a negative effect on both your work and home life.

Reading this book will guide you towards achieving enhanced wellbeing for greater productivity and overall happiness and steer you away from potential burnout. If you'd like to achieve your greatest ambition without the sacrifice of your health, wellbeing or relationships, then this is for you. You will have the ideal opportunity to reflect and take stock as I guide you through a selection of reflective practices before sharing a variety of wellbeing theories and techniques.

By the end of this book, you will feel emboldened and empowered to structure your working schedule in the most efficient way and to reap the rewards not only for your business, but also for your health, wellbeing and relationships. 'Burnout' will no longer be a barrier to your success.

The PROSPER model

I developed the PROSPER model to guide you through the seven key characteristics you will need to balance your working life with your health and wellbeing:

Purpose: Finding your purpose can help you become unstoppable. This clarity will help you shape your life accordingly by focusing on what really matters. Knowing your purpose will help you fuel your passion and live a value-based life. The PROSPER model will help you gain clarity on your passion, purpose and concept of happiness.

Resolve: Resolve is the steering mechanism that keeps you committed to staying on track to achieve your goals. It drives you to innovate and complete tasks. It is resolve that motivates you into action. The PROSPER model will help you explore overwhelm, procrastination and imposter syndrome to stay on track.

Opinion: At some level, every choice made has a positive or negative consequence. Making value-based decisions gives you clarity and removes much of the stress and pressure around choosing the correct path. The PROSPER model will help give you a deeper understanding of your own values and the importance of value-based decisions.

Strength of body and mind: Having a healthy body and mind is essential for everyday living and is something that we must nurture, just like an Olympic athlete or astronaut would to achieve optimal performance. The PROSPER model will provide insight into a wide range of techniques to develop a healthy mind and body, including sleep, physical activity, getting outdoors, mindfulness, meditation, gratitude and giving back.

Productivity: There is no denying that well-being and productivity go hand in hand. The PROSPER model will help you explore techniques to increase productivity, including ways to enhance your working environment, improve time management and build a harmonious support network.

Equilibrium: Balance means that your life will find its own equilibrium and ensure that when stressors and strains come along, they won't throw you off your direction. You'll be able to manage them and feel in control of your own destiny. The PROSPER model will help you achieve a work-life balance with techniques to switch off and maintain harmony.

Reward: Having something to look forward to increases your motivation and makes it easier to follow through with even the most challenging of tasks. Rewarding yourself is a great way to release positive emotions and adopt healthy behaviours. The PROSPER model will help you explore intrinsic and extrinsic award concepts, along with ways to apply them to the Stages of Change model.

Throughout this book I share accounts of my own journey, as well as case studies from successful entrepreneurs sharing the techniques that have worked for them and the challenges they have overcome.

In Part One, I will take you on a journey to explore the two P's: Prevention and Psychology. As we move through this section of the book and explore psychological theories, reflect on any key areas that you may wish to develop.

In Part Two, you will be guided through the first phase of the PROSPER model. This will provide insight into a range of wellbeing concepts and techniques, enabling you to choose which to implement into your daily life.

As you move on to Part Three, you will be guided through the final phase of the PROSPER model. This section will help you to consider how to implement the techniques shared in Part Two into your daily routine. I will also share additional factors to consider to maintain health and wellbeing while achieving your ambitions at work and at home.

By following the PROSPER model and adopting the techniques shared in this book, you will find your journey to entrepreneurial success not only rewarding, but your health, wellbeing and relationships will thrive too.

Enjoy the read.

PART ONE
PREVENTION AND PSYCHOLOGY

In Part One, I will take you on a journey to explore the two P's: Prevention and Psychology. To prevent burnout, you must first fully understand it. Chapter 1 explores burnout and stress in more detail, providing you with guidance to reflect on your own experience and behaviours when experiencing stress. As you progress to Chapter 2, three psychology theories are outlined. These theories provide insight into a range of lifestyle considerations that are believed to help build a healthy, happy and successful life. Use Part One to reflect on areas of your life that you may want to develop before you begin to explore the PROSPER model in Part Two of the book.

ONE
Prevention

This chapter provides insight into burnout and stress, including how to recognise it and ways to combat it. As no two people are the same, there's not a single solution. Immerse yourself in this chapter to gain a deeper understanding of your signs and symptoms, what is causing you to feel stressed and any negative responses you may have. Once you are aware of these, use the second section of the chapter to start identifying techniques to help you manage your stress effectively.

Understanding burnout

As an ambitious, hardworking entrepreneur, you may have found yourself working more hours than you had anticipated to make your ambitions a reality. This, combined with the day-to-day challenges of running a business, maintaining a social life and meeting other personal commitments, can be a juggling act. Get this wrong and the journey towards burnout can be all too easy.

To prevent burnout, you must first fully understand what it is and how it can manifest itself. In May 2018, the World Health Organization classified job 'burnout' as an occupational phenomenon. It defined burnout as a syndrome resulting from chronic workplace stress that has not been managed adequately.[1] Long hours and constant pressure to secure results can take their toll, even on the most resilient business owners. This work pressure, combined with the demands of daily life, can cause burnout if not sufficiently addressed.

Burnout can negatively impact your health, career and relationships. In the 1970s, Herbert Freudenberger described burnout as a severe stress condition that leads to severe physical, mental and emotional exhaustion.[2] It can leave you feeling as if you have nothing more to give and can no longer find joy in the things you once did. Day-to-day challenges and responsibilities that you normally deal with easily can feel like a mountain to climb or simply unachievable. If you're experiencing burnout, you may feel drained, pessimistic, isolated and hopeless. If left untreated, burnout can lead to serious physical and psychological illnesses such as depression, anxiety, heart disease and diabetes, so it's important to recognise it before it leads to serious implications.

CASE STUDY: CHARLOTTE

Charlotte has developed a way of dealing with burnout during the last two decades. She's owned a successful PR and marketing agency for fourteen years and has put enormous internal pressure on herself to achieve her goals.

Her first experience of burnout was when she was just seventeen years old. She was a promising Team GB athlete and a high-achieving student predicted to secure top grades in her A-levels. However, the pressure mounted and came to a head at a training camp in France. She suffered severe burnout, which led to her being wheelchair-bound. This gave rise to depression and she was forced to take a year out.

Charlotte has reflected on why she has a tendency to experience burnout. When she is focused on her goals, be it as a young athlete or when building her business, she gives everything she's got. The internal pressure she places on herself is often detrimental, not only to her health and wellbeing, but also to her relationships.

When setting up her business, she was so passionate and focused on making it work that her life was all work and no play. With no prior experience, she felt she had to give that 'little bit extra' to succeed. Working all hours, Charlotte was unable to dedicate time to her personal relationship and it broke down. After the split, she went on holiday to take a pause and regroup. It was during this break that she realised she had been working far too hard and had neglected other areas of her life that were just as important, if not more so, than her business. This included the relationship breakdown with her partner, but it had also impacted her health and wellbeing. She describes that holiday as a cathartic experience. It involved a lot of tears, emotions and realisations and taught her some important lessons about how she needed to

get her work-life balance more finely tuned
to succeed with both her business and her
life goals.

Continuously high levels of stress at home
or from internal pressures can have the same
result as work-induced burnout. Common
signs of burnout include:

1. **Exhaustion:** Lack of sleep and extreme
   tiredness can lead to additional symptoms
   such as irritability, headaches and
   impaired decision-making. Exhaustion can
   leave you without the energy to complete
   daily tasks, resulting in your workload
   piling up and stress levels increasing
   further.

2. **Overwhelm:** Experiencing emotional
   overwhelm can leave you feeling intense
   emotions that are difficult to manage.
   This can present itself as anxiety, worry,
   anger and irritability and can affect your
   self-esteem. All of these emotions can have
   a significant impact on the way you think,
   act and perform daily tasks.

3. **Detachment:** Emotionally detaching from
   the people around you may feel like a

way to avoid unwanted drama, anxiety or stress – particularly when you feel like you already have enough on your plate – but it's likely that this will ultimately have a negative impact on these relationships, causing further stress and upset.

4. **A negative outlook:** A person going through burnout may be struggling to feel optimistic. You may find that small challenges feel like mountains to climb, that people are conspiring against you, that the situation will never get any better and that there is no way out.

5. **Anxiety:** You may experience anxiety if you are worried or afraid, particularly about things that are going to happen, or may happen, in the future. It can affect you mentally, emotionally and physically.

Burnout and stress have similar signs and symptoms, but burnout is a result of chronic stress that has not been effectively managed. Unlike stress, burnout will not come and go and is likely to require professional help.

Understanding stress

As chronic stress can lead to burnout, it is essential that you learn how to recognise and manage stress effectively to help prevent burnout. The Mental Health Foundation describes stress as, 'The feeling of being overwhelmed or unable to cope with mental or emotional pressure.'[3] This can be a buildup of smaller, stressful situations or a substantial event such as a relationship breakdown, an illness or the death of a loved one.

It's important to remember that what constitutes 'stress' is unique to each individual. The same situation may make one person feel a level of pressure that helps to motivate them, while it may make another person feel stressed. While some pressure is normal and can even help you to perform well, it's important to remember that excessive stress can ultimately interfere with your productivity and performance, home life and relationships and impact your mental and physical health.

When we become stressed, our bodies produce high levels of cortisol – a hormone that triggers a 'fight or flight' response. This is an automatic physiological reaction to a stressful or fearful event perceived as a threat. The sympathetic nervous system is triggered and prepares the body to fight or flee. When in fight or flight response, your body may react with increased heart rate and blood pressure, pale or flushed skin and dilated pupils. You may also find yourself feeling tense or trembling and your memory may be affected.

Our fight or flight response plays a critical role in how we react to dangerous situations. This was particularly critical during periods when our ancestors were required to run from predators, but today, our fight or flight response can be triggered when it's not required, such as when we're running late in traffic or tackling a heavy workload. Frequent, inappropriate activation of the fight or flight response can lead to the body thinking it's constantly under attack and result in chronic stress. When chronic stress occurs, it can disrupt almost every system in your body, including the immune, digestive and reproductive systems. Chronic stress also increases the risk of heart attacks and strokes and can leave you more vulnerable to depression, anxiety and other mental health problems. Negative behaviours as a result of stress can include smoking, drugs, drinking in excess, gambling, compulsive spending, over-working and emotional eating.

Signs, symptoms and stressors

It's almost impossible to eliminate all stressors from our lives, but we can learn how to deal with them effectively and in a healthy manner to perform at our best. A 2020 review titled 'Stress and Well-being in Entrepreneurship: A Critical Review and Future Research Agenda' investigated entrepreneurial stress and its impact on subjective wellbeing. This systematic review found that stress was reciprocally linked to the performance of their business. It says, 'Entrepreneurs may experience stress as a function of their profession, but their perceived and experienced stress may also impact their ability to run a venture.'[4]

Now that you have an understanding of the impact of stress and burnout, it's helpful to get into the habit of checking in with yourself routinely each month. It's sometimes the case that individuals working under high pressure are so focused on achieving results that they neglect this vital practice, resulting in burnout sneaking up on them.

The symptoms of stress and burnout vary from person to person and aren't always easy to spot, so it's essential to take the time for self-analysis and realise when they are becoming a problem. Look out for physical warnings such as headaches, muscle tension, over-tiredness or feeling run down.

CASE STUDY: LOU

As a social entrepreneur, Lou has been a driving force in the charity sector for over twenty years. Like many entrepreneurs, she has experienced many highs and lows. One of her biggest challenges was when the Covid pandemic hit. As her business was based on face-to-face interaction, within an instant, one of the company's biggest USPs was taken away as lockdown was announced. It was also during this time that Lou's mum was sadly diagnosed with a terminal illness with only a few weeks left to live.

'I don't think I could ever articulate the level of stress and pressure I felt,' she says.

Lou needed to maintain her business to secure income for her family and herself, as well as her employees. Thankfully, her friends and colleagues went above and beyond to help give her some space, but during her return to work demands increased and Lou hit a wall.

'When you suffer grief, what people don't talk about is your ability to make decisions,' she says. 'Deciding what to have for tea became the most stressful thing ever.'

At this point, getting out of bed and showering became an achievement. Lou started using positive psychology techniques, where the ethos is to feel more in control of your behaviour.

'When you're at a crisis point and burned out, it's sometimes hard to understand what you're thinking and why you're thinking it. If you want to change your feelings, you've got two ways to do that: what you do and what you think,' Lou says.

She started by making a strategy of 'doing actions' such as getting out of bed, having a shower and walking on the beach. These 'doing actions' also included a range of coping mechanisms such as taking a walk with friends. The next step was to consider how her thoughts were having an impact, in particular her self-talk and the importance of challenging the narrative in her mind.

She says, 'I started to put more strategies around my negative thoughts. If I said something like, "I can't believe you're not out of bed yet," then my self-talk would say, "But you're obviously needing a rest. When you're ready, you'll get out of bed." By doing this, I could set a time limit, too.'

Identifying your signs and symptoms

The way that stress can creep up on you is incredibly dangerous. It is easy to get used to being stressed as it starts to become familiar, and even feel normal. You might not even notice how much it's affecting you and the heavy toll it's taking, so it's important to take stock and recognise any warning signs and symptoms of stress overload. The signs and symptoms of stress can present themselves physically, mentally, emotionally and in the way that we behave. A few examples are listed below:

Physically:

- Headaches
- Stomach ache
- Sweaty palms
- Difficulty sleeping or sleeping too much
- Nausea
- Frequent colds or flu

Mentally:

- Memory problems
- Racing thoughts
- Poor judgement
- Lack of creativity
- Constant worrying
- Difficulty making decisions

Emotionally:

- Irritability
- Feeling anxious
- Moodiness
- Anger
- Feeling overwhelmed
- Unhappiness or depression

Behaviour:

- Avoiding people
- Being judgemental

- Drinking / smoking more

- Taking drugs

- Procrastination

- Nervous habits

TASK: Identifying stress symptoms

Use a piece of paper or a notebook to make a list of all your signs and symptoms under these four headings:

- Physically
- Mentally
- Emotionally
- My behaviour

Each time you experience the signs and symptoms that you have listed, stop and consider what is causing you to act or feel this way.

Identifying your stressors

When you're feeling stressed, it's important to understand what the root cause could be. A heavy workload, long hours, poor work-life balance, feeling a lack of control or dealing with a situation that's emotionally draining are a few examples. Taking some time to identify where your stressors are stemming from will help you zone in on what factors you can and can't control.

If you're struggling to put your finger on exactly what causes you to feel stressed, try keeping a diary over the next two to four weeks to identify any trends in situations that cause you the most stress. Make a note of your thoughts and feelings, as well as any other key information you remember about the people and circumstances. By doing so, you can start to look at what you can proactively change and what you need to let go of.

TASK: Identifying stress triggers

Make a list of everything that is causing you to feel anxious or stressed. Sort the possible reasons for your stress into two columns:

1. Those with a practical solution, for example, scheduling time to meet a work deadline or recruiting a new employee to share your workload.
2. Those you can't do anything about, for example, current affairs or the opinions of others.

For everything listed in the first column, start to make a plan on how you will act on each one. Try to release the worry of those in the second column and let them go.

Improving your ability to handle stress

The next step is to find the right tools and techniques to not only help you to effectively manage stress, but to help you thrive. Throughout this book, I share a wide range of concepts for you to consider and try as you wish. Remember, everyone is different. What works for one person may not work for another, so keep an open mind and see what works for you. There are four areas that are key contributors to help manage stress effectively:

1. **A strong support network:** A strong support network can act as a significant shield against stress. Having people that you can rely on and open up to about work and life's pressures can help reduce stress and overwhelm and provide peace of mind. Not having a strong support network can feel lonely and isolating, increasing your risk of stress.

2. **A positive outlook:** Your outlook on life and its challenges can make a significant difference in your ability to manage stress. If you're generally more optimistic, and you embrace change and any upcoming challenges then it's likely that you're better equipped to manage potentially stressful situations. As discussed in Lou's case study, we have the ability to challenge our thoughts and self-talk.

3. **Emotional intelligence:** By recognising and managing your emotions you can apply techniques to feel calm and relaxed when feeling negative emotions such as anger or sadness. Without this understanding, it's more likely that you will become agitated and stressed and less able to communicate how you're feeling with the people around you.

4. **A sense of control:** When you're stressed it can feel like things are running out of control. On the flip side, when you feel confident that you're able to influence a chain of events and persevere through challenges, this sense of control can make it easier to handle stress along the way. The more you know about a situation and the greater the level of confidence you

have in tackling it, the greater sense of control you will have.

Instant stress-busting activities

A useful technique is to have a list of instant stress-busting activities. This list should consist of activities that you can apply there and then if you're feeling stressed or at points throughout the day as you start to notice your signs and symptoms. It's important that these activities help you to feel good. For example, think about the emotions watching a film might evoke – will it leave you feeling relaxed, calm and uplifted?

TASK: Choose stress-busting activities

Make a list of ten instant stress-busting activities that you can carry out the next time you're feeling stressed. Examples include:

- Listening to an uplifting podcast
- Going for a walk
- Watching something that makes you laugh
- Exercising or dancing
- Catching up with a supportive friend
- Meditating

- Taking a relaxing bath
- Practising mindfulness
- Listening to uplifting music
- Giving someone a hug

Relaxing through the breath

When you feel stressed, your breathing patterns can change as part of your fight or flight response. Small, shallow breaths can overtake the natural rhythm of breathing from the diaphragm, which can prolong the feelings of anxiety and worsen any physical symptoms. Fortunately, you have the ability to override this. By slowing down your breath in a gentle and consistent way, you can calm the nervous system that controls the body's automatic functions. This can also support lowered blood pressure and heart rate, reduced levels of stress and increased immune function. Research shows that when practised regularly, there is reduced activity in the sympathetic nervous system (also known as the 'fight or flight' response).[5] Here are two breathing exercises that can aid with reducing anxiety and help you relax.

Diaphragmatic breathing: Your diaphragm is a muscle that helps you to breathe, but when breathing normally we don't often use our lungs to full capacity. Place one hand on your belly and one hand on your chest and breathe normally. Notice which hand naturally rises and falls more. For most people, this is the hand on the chest, where the breath is predominantly held in the top of the lungs. During diaphragmatic breathing, you will feel more movement in the stomach as you consciously use your diaphragm to take deep breaths to use your lungs at greater capacity.

Take a deep breath in slowly through the nose until you feel a little resistance in the chest. The diaphragm will continue to contract and move downwards to pull the air into the bottom of the lungs. You will feel your belly rise as it relaxes and the sides of your lungs expand. Pause for a moment before slowly releasing the breath through the mouth, as if you are blowing out a candle. As the breath is released, the diaphragm moves up and the navel moves towards the spine. As you repeat this exercise, start to focus on relaxing your body. Continue breathing like this for 3–5 minutes.

Alternate nostril breathing: This simple exercise is a yoga breathing technique (also known as Nadi Shodhana Pranayama) which aims to balance energy flow. During this breathing exercise, you will need to use your thumb to close one nostril and your ring finger to close the other. Using your right hand, close the two fingers between your thumb and ring finger.

Sitting in a comfortable, upright position, lift your right hand and close your right nostril with your thumb. Inhale through the left nostril for 3–5 seconds. Momentarily close your nose with your ring finger. Keeping your ring finger on your left nostril, remove your thumb and breathe out of your right nostril for 3–5 seconds. Keeping your hand in the same position, breathe in for 4 seconds through your right nostril. Momentarily close your nose with your thumb, release your ring finger and repeat the exercise. Repeat this procedure five times.

TASK: Breathing exercises

Dedicate just a few minutes a day to carry out a calming breathing exercise, such as those listed above. It's great to end a long, busy day by relaxing through these exercises, but equally, it could be done at the start of the day for a calm and collected mind, or at any point during the day where you feel you need for time out from work.

Be sure to check in with your doctor if you have any medical concerns regarding these exercises and discontinue if you feel discomfort, panic and hyperventilation.

Summary

Burnout is a physiological and psychological consequence of chronic stress. It can lead to a range of long- and short-term health conditions such as heart disease, anxiety and depression. To prevent burnout, it's key to recognise:

- Your signs and symptoms
- What is causing you stress
- Any negative responses to stress
- Techniques to help you manage stress effectively

TWO
Psychology

This chapter focuses on three psychology theories: positive psychology, Maslow's Hierarchy of Needs and Rogers' Self-Actualisation, or Humanistic, Theory. Each theory provides insight into a range of life-style considerations that are believed to help build a healthy, happy and successful life. Use this chapter to reflect on areas of your life that you may want to further develop before we embark upon the PROSPER model.

The first theory, positive psychology, explores the impact a positive mindset can have on achieving a fulfilling life. Techniques include acknowledging personal strengths, celebrating successes, embracing positive relationships and implementing positive lifestyle choices for good health and wellbeing.

The second theory, Maslow's Hierarchy of Needs, highlights five building blocks of needs that, if achieved at each stage, can enhance your feelings of achievement and fulfilment.

The final theory is about understanding who you are, who you would ideally like to be in the future, and who you perceive yourself to be currently. Rogers' Humanistic Theory provides insight into developing congruence between your ideal self and your self-image to achieve greater self-esteem.

Positive psychology

The founder of positive psychology, Martin Seligman, grew frustrated with psychology's attention to the negative and a relatively limited focus on happiness, wellbeing and flourishing. He pioneered a revolution through the positive psychology movement which focuses on emotions such as happiness, kindness and hope, and character strengths, including self-esteem and how such traits can be applied to everyday activities for a meaningful life.[6]

Positive psychology is intended to complement, enrich and understand human experience rather than replace or eliminate disadvantage or suffering. Its theories explain that happiness, character strengths and positive relationships act as a buffer against setbacks. It's essential to feel engaged and to be able to draw meaning from our work or to be working towards a purpose. According to University of Michigan professor Christopher Peterson, research in the field has proved that living a good life can be taught and for the most part, people are happy and generally resilient. Good days have three factors in common: autonomy, competence and connection to others.[7]

The benefits of positive psychology

- **Increased confidence and awareness of personal strengths:** Applying specific positive psychology practices can help you identify strengths that might have otherwise been missed. Focusing on strengths can help increase confidence, enthusiasm and resilience.

- **Improved relationships:** Studies have shown that the strength of our relationships plays a significant role in our levels of happiness.[8] The way in which you communicate with others is vital in building good relationships. Focusing on positive, yet truthful and authentic, communication can be of significant benefit to you and those you communicate with.

- **Increased focus on health and wellbeing:** Actively practising positive psychology techniques on a regular basis is one way of actively encouraging healthy behaviour change. Research has shown significant health benefits, such as cardiovascular recovery after a stressful event can be sped up through positive emotions.[9] Another example is the immune function, which can be boosted by mindfulness meditation.

- **Focus on success:** Positive psychology techniques can help shape the way you think about events in your life. This can provide you with the best possible mindset to overcome fear and challenges and to be confident and persistent in the pursuit of success.

- **Stronger communities:** Whether it's in the workplace or at home, positive psychology techniques can be practised by all to increase a positive environment. Those that carry out acts of kindness, for example, not only get a boost in wellbeing, but are more appreciated and accepted by their peers. Happiness is contagious and those surrounded by happy friends, colleagues and family members are more likely to be happy themselves. In the workplace, if employees are happy, it can also improve how they respond to customers. The knock-on effect of all of this is an environment where individuals feel cared for and are able to thrive.

FOLLOW-UP WITH LOU

As Lou continues on her entrepreneurial journey, she has found a number of techniques to help her along the way. She says, 'I take action to not be around anything that I feel might influence my mood in a negative way, such as regularly deactivating my social media and keeping away from anything that might zap my energy.'

Another technique Lou finds useful is challenging the difference between perception and reality. She says, 'For example, do I feel that

that person has been rude to me, or is it just my perception? What's the reality? Actually, that person might be dealing with something. Is someone mad at me as I've not got back to their email, or was it just my perception and the reality is they understand that I'm all over the place at the moment and that's OK.'

Applying positive psychology to everyday activities

There are many ways in which we can apply positive psychology to everyday life. This includes practising gratitude each day, checking in on negative self-talk and carrying out simple acts of kindness (read more about these techniques in Chapter 6). Here are two positive psychology tasks that you can do right away.

TASK 1: A letter of self-compassion

When confronted with failures, mistakes or shortcomings, it's important to treat yourself with compassion, care and concern.

Try and set aside thirty minutes of your day to complete this task. Make sure that you're in a comfortable and relaxing space that allows you to fully focus on the task at hand.

First, choose a personal aspect of yourself that you dislike, that could do with improvement or that you are self-critical about. Write in detail how this perceived negative trait makes you feel. What images, emotions and memories does this evoke?

Next, imagine someone you trust and respect who loves you unconditionally. It could be a friend, family member or a romantic partner. This person recognises both your positive and negative traits. If you ever let them down, they are always forgiving and understanding and will always help you find your way to grow. Write a letter to yourself from this person's perspective:

- How do they see you from their perspective?

- What do they say to you?

- How do they encourage you?

- How do they support you to make changes in your life?

Once you've drafted your letter, put it aside for fifteen minutes. Return to it and absorb the words and meaning of the letter. Feel the emotions and the natural high it gives you when you read the words of encouragement, support, compassion and acceptance. Each time you are feeling down or negative about your life or work or lacking in self-belief and need a boost, read your letter, absorb it, embrace the positive vibes it gives you, and most importantly of all, accept yourself in the way that your trusted friend or family member accepts you. This is the first step to change.

TASK 2: Treasure box

Look for a box that you find appealing – something that makes you want to explore it. If you're feeling creative, perhaps add some personal touches. (If you have children, this is a great activity for them to try, too.) Once your chosen treasure box is ready, it's time to start collecting happy memories, thoughts and items that bring you joy. Whenever something makes you feel happy, write it down, take a picture or draw it and then pop it into your treasure box. The next time you find yourself feeling unhappy, take out the treasure box and reflect on each item and the happiness it brings you.

Taking time out to focus on these individual memories acts as a trigger to release the positivity hormone, dopamine (also known as the 'happy hormone'). For example, when you look at a photograph of your favourite holiday destination, it brings back memories from when you were there, what you did, who you were with and so on. These positive memories can reset your brain into thinking positively.

Maslow's Hierarchy of Needs

Psychologist Abraham Maslow wanted to find out what makes life purposeful for people. He developed a theory that suggests people are motivated to satisfy five basic needs. Arranged in a hierarchy, Maslow suggests that the first stage of needs must be satisfied before seeking to satisfy the next level. This pattern should continue until all five stages are satisfied. The triangular diagram below gives a clear illustration of the five levels:

1. Physiological needs: food, air, water, sleep, warmth, shelter, reproduction

2. Security needs: protection, stability, law, free from fear, financial security

3. Love and belonging needs: friendship, intimate relationships, family

4. Esteem needs: self-esteem, confidence, achievement, respect from others

5. Self-actualisation needs: meeting one's full potential in life

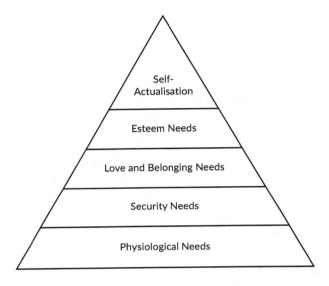

Maslow's Hierarchy of Needs

Maslow argued that the failure to meet the first four stages of the hierarchy of needs, also known as deficiency needs, could lead to ill-health and even death. For example, physiological needs such as clean water, good food and shelter are essential for life. When security needs such as receiving a stable income or being free from fear are not met, then stress or anxiety can occur. At the top of the pyramid is self-actualisation, where an individual will fulfil their own potential. As the GoodTherapy blog explains, 'The necessary components of self-actualization vary from person to person. A scientist may be self-actualized when able to complete research in a chosen field. A father might be self-actualized when able to competently care for his children.'[10]

Maslow studied and recorded a number of people from history that he believed had reached self-actualisation, including theoretical physicist Albert Einstein, humanitarian Eleanor Roosevelt, Nobel Peace Prize recipient Albert Schweitzer and 17th century philosopher Baruch Spinoza.[11] According to Maslow, some of the characteristics that define self-actualised individuals include:

- Authenticity

- An appreciation of life

- A core purpose

- Seeing the 'bigger picture' and untroubled by small things

- Living in the present moment

- Not thinking they are perfect

Rogers' Humanistic Theory

Carl Rogers, a humanistic psychologist, believed that given the right conditions, a person could grow and blossom to reach their full potential. According to Rogers, 'The good life is a process, not a state of being. It is a direction not a destination.'[12] His self-concept theory is basically a personal analysis of how you view yourself. It can be influenced by your childhood and how society perceives you and can be broken down into three aspects:

1. **True self:** This is who you really are from an objective perspective.

2. **Ideal self:** This is who you would ideally like to be, or who you are striving towards being. Your ideal self can adapt as your goals and ambitions evolve over time.

3. **Self-image:** This is how you perceive yourself as a human being in society, for example, successful or unsuccessful, healthy or unhealthy, kind or unkind. It's what you see when you look in the mirror and relates to self-esteem.

Rogers believed that for a person to achieve self-actualisation, they must be in a state of congruence – a term used to describe an overlap of the self-image and ideal self. The greater the overlap, the more congruence you have in life and the greater your self-esteem.

Reaching self-actualisation would allow someone to become 'fully functioning', which includes trusting yourself to make correct decisions, having a high regard of self, enjoying the present moment, living in harmony and being able to adapt your life in accordance to open feedback.

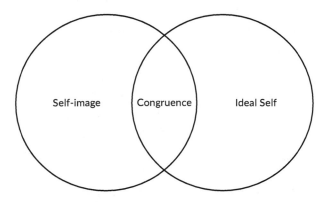

Rogers' Self-Actualisation Theory

Rogers explained that individuals living in an environment with openness, opportunities for self-disclosure, acceptance and empathy are more likely to hold congruent views of themselves that align to how the rest of the world sees them. As Dr Saul McLeod explains,

'The closer our self-image and ideal self are to each other, the more consistent or congruent we are and the higher our sense of self-worth. A person is said to be in a state of incongruence if some of the totality of their experience is unacceptable to them and is denied or distorted in the self-image.'[13]

TASK: Considering your self

Take a few minutes to think about the questions below:

- **Your ideal self:** What would you ideally like to be/what are you currently striving towards being?

- **Your self-image:** How do you perceive yourself as a human being in society? What do you see when you look in the mirror?

- **The overlap:** How big is the overlap between your ideal self and self-image? Is this is something that you can work on further?

Summary

Psychology is important when it comes to maintaining your health and wellbeing and to prevent burnout. In this chapter we have explored three theories: positive psychology, Maslow's Hierarchy of Needs and Rogers' Humanistic Theory. Keeping those theories in mind, reflect on these questions:

- Could positive psychology techniques be applied to your everyday activities to create greater happiness and meaning?

- Which of Maslow's five needs are being fulfilled and which need further development?

- Would you like to be more congruent, and if so, how could you achieve this?

PART TWO
PHASE ONE OF THE PROSPER MODEL

In Part Two of this book, you will be guided through the first phase of the PROSPER model (Purpose, Resolve, Opinion and Strength). We will explore key principles to help you:

- Reach your goals by exploring your passion, purpose and happiness

- Become unstoppable by addressing overwhelm, procrastination and imposter syndrome

- Stay on track by checking in on your values, value-based decisions and authenticity

- Maintain a healthy mind and body by exploring the benefits of a good night's sleep, regular physical activity, getting outdoors, mindfulness, gratitude and positivity and giving back

THREE
Purpose

This chapter focuses on **purpose** and includes concepts for finding your passion and exploring happiness. The clarity gained from finding your purpose will help you shape your life by focusing on what really matters. Knowing your purpose will help fuel your passion to reach your goals.

Passion

Why is passion important?

Having passion to achieve what you do is one of the best ways to maintain motivation. When challenges crop up, passion can give you the determination to overcome obstacles and go above and beyond to achieve your goals. Passion correlates with success.

As a teenager, I wasn't content with my choice of subjects upon leaving school. I chose those that I was good at and that I thought would help me on my way to a great career, but they weren't subjects that I felt overly passionate about – mathematics, biology and physics. Looking back, it seems unusual for a sixteen-year-old to be questioning their passion and purpose, but I believe the loss of three family members and one of my best friends in a short space of time had a significant influence on my decision to find something more meaningful and *exude* happiness. I made the decision to change college and study a whole new range of subjects based on what I felt most passionate about. I reflected on when I felt my happiest, what part of this gave me joy, and whether I was good at it. The answer was simple: it was when I was dancing and being creative. Although it can be incredibly difficult to successfully break into the Arts and I knew the road ahead would be a challenging one, I knew I had to follow this path.

I achieved a first-class honours degree in Contemporary Dance as well as dancing for motion capture film, TV and Bollywood. As a student working part-time, my hourly pay was five times more as a dance teacher than in my previous part-time role as a sales assistant. The best feeling was that none of this even felt like work. I loved every minute of it. Upon graduating, I used my passion for dance and enthusiasm for meaningful work to start my first company, Nuvo Wellbeing, a multi-award-winning social enterprise that encourages increased fitness levels, personal development and healthy lifestyle choices – helping people and communities to feel positive, be active and live well.

CASE STUDY: ALICE

Alice started her first business at the age of twenty-three while working as a cover teacher in a high school. Her mum gave her £90, which she used to purchase a pack of dresses to sell online. The dresses sold quickly and Alice continued to reinvest, purchasing and selling more dresses. Although initially drawn into setting up a business to provide an additional source of income, Alice found that she had a passion for creativity. With her mum by her side, the duo went on to grow the business. Within six years, they had a turnover of £25 million. With Alice focusing on creative aspects such as marketing and buying and her mum managing the business and its finances, they were able to create a thriving business. Alice found that working at a senior level could draw her away from the creative aspect of the business at times, but in the process of setting up her second e-commerce company she made a conscious decision to continue in her area of passion, in which she excels.

Finding your passion

As well as finding something that you enjoy doing, finding your passion involves understanding what motivates you. The key is to understand why you want to accomplish something, not what you need to do to accomplish it. For some people, this could be solving complex problems through innovation or helping others.

As an ex-professional dancer, I've always had a significant interest in health and wellbeing. I was shocked to find that life expectancy in many deprived areas of the UK was between eight to ten years lower than the national average.[14] Associated diseases such as diabetes, cardiovascular disease and obesity were all significantly higher than the national average. Local statistics also demonstrated that sedentary lifestyles in both adults and children were increasingly high, but with few opportunities to access local, affordable physical activities, how could local communities make lifestyle changes to improve their health and wellbeing? It was then that I knew I could combine my interest in health and wellbeing with my passion for helping others to make a difference. Just like dance had helped me, I knew it could help others too.

TASK: Finding your passion

If you're interested in exploring your areas of passion further, start by answering these four questions:

1. Is there something that you really enjoy doing?
2. What do you spend your time reading or learning about?

3. What would your close friends and family say your passion was?

4. Is this aligned to your business or job role?

Remember, only you can write your story.

Why is purpose important?

Finding your purpose can help you become unstoppable. There are many benefits to understanding your purpose, including:

1. **Unlocking your true potential:** Following your life purpose can give you the ability to unlock your true potential, including your natural talents. This might be something that you have already been doing on a daily basis or something you haven't yet fully explored.

2. **Igniting your passion:** Have you ever found yourself successfully climbing the career ladder or building a business, but still feeling dissatisfied? This often indicates a lack of meaning or purpose. Finding your purpose can ignite your passion and help you feel fully aligned.

3. **Gaining clarity on what is, and isn't, important:** Understanding your purpose can give you clarity on what is important to you to fulfil your goals, but also what isn't important. This can save time, energy and resources.

4. **Unlocking abundance:** Performing work that you love and that is aligned to your purpose will lead to success. Money will flow to you as a by-product of this success.

5. **Achieving success:** We all have our own concept of what 'success' looks like and it generally changes over time, but finding and following your purpose is a sure way for you to achieve whatever you see it as.

6. **Building positive relationships:** While working on your purpose, it's likely that you will naturally come across like-minded individuals that you can share passions with and offer support to one another along the way.

7. **Living a life of meaning:** Finding your purpose can give life a greater meaning. Contributing to something bigger than yourself improves positive feelings such as happiness and fulfilment.

8. **Improving health and wellbeing:**
   Fulfilling your purpose will give you a
   sense of satisfaction, which can improve
   happiness. This can have a positive impact
   on both your physical and mental health
   and wellbeing.

Feelings of lingering dissatisfaction and not
being in sync with your inner self are common experiences for those who have not yet
found their purpose. Sometimes your purpose
can be right in front of you, but there could
be something blocking you from seeing it.
An example is when someone who is drawn
to volunteering in a particular field or sector
feels more aligned to this kind of work than to
their day job.

Purpose is a deep underlying sense of peace –
a gut feeling that you're on the right path and
the challenges you face along the way won't
discourage you from continuing on this road.
It's important not to mistake happiness for
purpose. Happiness naturally comes and goes
throughout life experiences and situations.
Some people go through life questioning their
purpose on a regular basis, while others have
successfully identified their purpose but have

made conscious decisions to follow different routes.

When you start your business as an entrepreneur, your purpose may be at the forefront of your mind and fuelled by your passion, but various factors along your journey such as changes at home, demands from investors or new opportunities can pull you off track. It's important to check in every now and again to make sure your decisions and your business purpose remain fully aligned. As well as supporting important decisions, this will help drive the business in the right direction, while supporting your personal health and happiness.

After eight years of growing and developing Nuvo Wellbeing, I started to get 'itchy feet'. The organisation was carrying out amazing work and changing lives, but within this time I had also grown and developed. No longer a graduate fresh out of university, I had experienced some of life's greatest pressures while growing a business and my passion for wellbeing had become even greater. Within my network of entrepreneurs, social entrepreneurs and senior leaders, individuals would open up to me about their challenges, seek support to create greater balance and ask for guidance to over-come a particular obstacle. Putting the needs of employees, stakeholders and customers before my own became the norm. Looking back, it's hard to believe that the organisation I founded was helping hundreds of people every week to improve their wellbeing, yet I was at times neglecting my own. If you can relate to this, then an important question to ask yourself is, 'Where would my company be if I was unable to run it?' I have found that this question often puts into perspective the absolute need to not only prioritise wellness, but to use wellbeing techniques to help prosper in all aspects of life. With this in mind, I began creating OptiMe, a digital tool that could help people from every sector of an organisation to manage their own wellbeing and learn how to thrive.

OptiMe

OptiMe is a proven approach to health and wellbeing in the workplace. It is designed to:

1. Reduce stress (so that burnout doesn't become a concern)

2. Promote easy methods to improve physical and mental health

3. Accelerate team productivity and encourage members to stay engaged

4. Influence positive, collaborative relationships among colleagues in the workplace and working remotely

5. Work with the HR department to instil an empowered culture

If you are interested in learning more about OptiMe, please visit http://bethanyainsley.com.

Happiness

Happiness is defined as an emotional state characterised by feelings of joy, satisfaction, contentment and fulfilment.[15] Research has shown that happy people are healthier, live longer and enjoy a higher quality of life. It's unrealistic to think that we should feel happy in every moment of our life. In fact, it's healthy to experience and recognise emotions such as sadness, fear and anger. Emotionally healthy people are in control of their thoughts, feelings and behaviours. They keep problems in perspective and bounce back from challenges.

Your definition of happiness is likely to differ to others, as it's based on your personal perspective. Scientists have usefully described happiness as having two components: experiencing more positive feelings than negative ones on a daily basis and how satisfied you feel with areas of your life that you consider important such as work, relationships and home life. These aspects are usually referred to as pleasure and meaning. Research shows that happy people are more productive at work, build better relationships and help others.[16]

Approximately 50% of your happiness is controlled by your genetic makeup, 40% is controlled by thoughts, actions and behaviours, and only 10% is controlled by your circumstances. Often quoted by positive psychologists, these figures support the theory that a large proportion of your happiness is within your control.[17] They also highlight the importance of developing a happiness toolkit, which can give you a range of helpful practices to further develop this area of your life.

Developing a happiness toolkit

A happiness toolkit is a list of powerful action tools to help build your happiest life. See how many of these points you can apply to your daily life:

1. **Practise gratitude:** At the beginning and end of each day, think of three to five things that you're grateful for. This will put you in the right mindset for the day ahead and help you fall asleep feeling positive. (Read more about this in Chapter 6.)

2. **Practise optimism:** Try to see the best in situations, people and circumstances. Make it an intention to picture positive outcomes. Challenge negative thoughts with perception vs reality and practise kinder self-talk.

3. **Surround yourself with supporting, positive people:** Being around people that match or raise your energy can give you a boost in feel-good hormones. Having the support of good people can help you overcome challenges and drive motivation and ambition on your road to success.

4. **Don't compare yourself to others:** If you find yourself comparing yourself to others and it's having a negative effect on your self-esteem or mental wellbeing, then change the focus back to your

DON'T BURN OUT, STAND OUT

own life. You may need to take a break from social media or re-evaluate who you're following. Recognise your own achievements and the things you like about yourself. When you become happy and fulfilled in your own life, it doesn't matter what others are doing.

5. **Live in the present:** Try to stop worrying about everything that needs to be done tomorrow or the week ahead. Instead, create an effective plan forward and then enjoy the present moment.

6. **Learn to accept what you can't change:** If something is out of your control, then learn to accept that and try to let it go. If something can be changed, then make a list of actions that you can start implementing.

7. **Learn to manage stress effectively:** As detailed in Chapter 1, stress plays a pivotal role in our health and wellbeing. Stress can disrupt the brain's ability to modulate feel-good chemicals of serotonin, norepinephrine and dopamine.

8. **Give back:** Helping others boosts feelings of happiness and optimism. It can also encourage recipients to repeat good deeds,

contributing to a positive community. There are many ways in which you can give back, for example, volunteering, raising money for a good cause or simply being kind to others. (Read more about this in Chapter 6.)

9. **Get active:** Ensure that you're moving around as much as possible, especially if your work involves being sedentary. Choose exercise that you enjoy and will continue to engage in even on busy days or when you're not quite feeling like it.

10. **Spend time in nature:** Spending time in nature or even viewing nature scenes can help reduce negative emotions such as anger and stress. It can also help your physical health by lowering blood pressure. Nature can help you feel great, so get outdoors and make the most of your local park, countryside or coast.

By implementing these techniques into your daily life, you can gain greater control over your emotions, behaviours and thought process, helping to keep problems in perspective, bounce back from challenges and choose happiness. The next two tasks can be practised at any point throughout this journey, but they could also be a great way to get you started, so why not try them today.

TASK 1: Practising gratitude

Close your eyes and take a few moments to think about someone influential in your life. Now write down everything that you appreciate about them. When your list is complete, read your list to them over the phone or in person. (If that's not possible, perhaps share it with them by email or via a private messaging app.) Finally, reflect on how this exercise made you feel.

TASK 2: Happiness journal

Spend five minutes writing about one positive experience that happened to you in the past twenty-four hours. Include what happened, how it made you feel and what you are grateful for. Reliving a positive experience like this will extend the feel-good factor and give you the time to really appreciate the experience.

Summary

Following your passion and purpose will help you to reach your own meaningful goals, while understanding how to increase happiness in your life will make the journey both pleasurable and fulfilling. In this chapter we've explored passion, purpose and happiness. Keeping those topics in mind, reflect on these questions:

- What are your burning passions?

- What activities or causes do you feel most aligned with?

- Which techniques from the happiness toolkit will you implement into your daily life?

FOUR
Resolve

Resolve is the steering mechanism that keeps you committed to staying on track to achieve your goals. It drives you to innovate and complete tasks. It is resolve that motivates you into action. In this chapter, we look at techniques to tackle overwhelm, procrastination and imposter syndrome to help you stay on track and achieve your goals.

Overwhelm

The mind of an entrepreneur is often required to run at a fast pace to make the most of opportunities, overcome obstacles and learn from setbacks. While most of the time you're achieving great things and making an impact on the world, it's also normal to occasionally feel overwhelmed, uncomfortable and unbalanced. As an entrepreneur, it's essential that you learn to deal with overwhelm to remain resilient as your business continues to grow and to overcome any challenges which may lie ahead. Next time you're feeling overwhelmed, consider trying one of these strategies to help bring you back into alignment:

1. **Write it down:** Taking some time to write everything down can help release your mind from ruminating thoughts, emotions and tasks that need to be completed. Seeing everything in front of you (either on paper or digitally) can help you organise your thoughts and your to-do list. I find that having a to-do list helps me to stay focused and ticking off the tasks as I go gives me a sense of accomplishment. The key is to ensure that your to-do list is

realistic and you provide enough time to effectively and efficiently tackle each task.

2. **Take a moment:** Sometimes, you just need to take a moment to pause and reset. Take this time to focus on yourself, move into a space where you can relax and practise one of your stress-busting activities. This could be going for a walk to get some fresh air, listening to a meditation exercise or just having a mindful cup of tea without distractions. Come back to your work once you're feeling refreshed.

3. **Delegate:** As an entrepreneur, you're in control of countless decisions and numerous tasks. As your workload builds, it's essential to delegate to help keep your workload manageable, to continue delivering at a high quality and to maintain your wellbeing. This could be offloading some work to an employee, outsourcing tasks such as marketing or looking at ways to automate through online systems.

4. **Ask for help:** If you're feeling overwhelmed, it can help to speak to someone who will understand what you're going through. If you've got a

mentor, business partner or supportive friends who have been in a similar situation, they are likely to be able to offer support and guidance. Pick up the phone and start a conversation with one of them.

Procrastination

Like most entrepreneurs, I imagine you're juggling several projects, numerous daily tasks and plenty of new ideas. Skirting around any of these without making progressive steps forward can slow down your success and even become detrimental to your business. Procrastination is one of the biggest entrepreneurial challenges. It is something that even the most successful people are challenged with, but they have learned how to recognise and manage it – something we should all be striving for.

Consistency and discipline form habits, so stay focused and avoid unnecessary distractions. Think about the sense of accomplishment you get from ticking off all the tasks on your to-do list at the end of the day. It feels great, doesn't it? Why does it sometimes feel so difficult, then? Four reasons that I hear on a regular basis are:

1. **Something else is more enticing:** Imagine that there's a task that you've been putting off for a while. The longer you leave it, the worse it feels. As this feeling grows, you put every other task above it – even those less important. This pattern continues and the task becomes an even greater challenge in your mind, with stress levels increasing. If you find yourself in a position where you're putting off a particular task, then do it first. Chances are it isn't as bad as you'd anticipated and you'll feel a whole lot better once you can mark it off as complete.

   If you work with your phone next to you or you have notifications on your work computer, then social media, news, messages and emails are all potential distractions. If it's not essential, then try keeping your mobile phone out of sight so you don't automatically reach for it or get distracted by notifications popping up. Also take some time to consider whether notifications on your work computer are essential or can be reduced.

Think about how you can make work more exciting. Playing music can be a great motivator if you find tracks that give you a boost. Also try rewarding yourself when you've achieved a goal. It doesn't have to be anything big – just something that makes you feel good (for me, this would probably be a piece of cake!).

2. **Struggling to get started:** Often, the biggest challenge is getting started in the first place. The longer you put something off, the worse it's going to feel to get going. To help with this, make sure that you have all of the information you need and then break the task down into small, manageable chunks. Focus on one task at a time and set a realistic timeframe to get each one completed.

3. **There isn't enough time to get it done:** Studies have shown that in most cases, a person will complete a task in the amount of time that they have allocated to it.[18] If they have allocated too much time, then they will still use the full amount of time to complete the task. If they allocate too little time, they will become overwhelmed. The trick is to allocate just the right amount of time and complete the task in

short bursts to maintain concentration and maximise productivity.

4. **Feeling too tired to focus:** Tiredness can have a significant impact on your productivity and how you feel (I share more findings on this in Chapter 6). I always tell my clients that it's important to listen to your body, so if you're feeling tired and struggling to concentrate, then take a break. The purpose of the break is to rest and recharge, so don't be tempted to check your work emails or respond to calls. During this rest time, practise activities that will leave you recharged and ready to refocus, such as having a power nap, practising meditation or getting some fresh air. Once you return to your work, remember to stay hydrated to keep energy levels up, avoid distractions that can zap your energy and take regular breaks to recharge.

If you're feeling fatigued on a regular basis, then it's a good idea to analyse what the root cause could be. For example, reaching for a cup of coffee may seem like the most helpful thing to do to give you another boost in energy, but a high caffeine intake could be affecting your sleep and result in tiredness during the day. The Royal College of Psychiatrists recommends that you stop drinking caffeine by mid-afternoon as it lingers in the body for several hours.[19] If you're tired on a regular basis through difficulty sleeping, then try cutting out caffeine completely.

As well as procrastinating at work, it's easy to find yourself procrastinating at home. Putting off house chores, sorting through your home admin or having a challenging conversation with a friend are all examples of things we tend to procrastinate. It's important to remember that procrastinating and putting off things that need to be done can cause increased stress. The task will linger in the back of your mind while the problem exacerbates, the deadline gets shorter and shorter or a vital opportunity is missed.

Overcoming procrastination

If you tend to struggle with procrastination (either regularly or even just from time to time), then these three steps can help you gain a deeper understanding on when you procrastinate, what triggers it and how you can better manage it:

1. Start by analysing your current behaviour:

    - When was the last time you found yourself procrastinating?

    - What was the task that you had to complete?

    - How did this task make you feel?

    - What did you find yourself doing instead of the allocated task and how did this make you feel?

2. Once you've identified potential triggers for procrastination (for example, a work presentation that you're not looking forward to or a difficult conversation with a relative), devise a carefully considered plan that removes any opportunities to procrastinate. This could be working in another room away from distractions such as the TV or your partner. Remind yourself that by getting the task at hand completed, you will feel a sense of accomplishment.

3. Reward yourself for completing the task without procrastinating. Overcoming procrastination is something that requires ongoing practice, so be patient, persevere and acknowledge any positive behaviour changes.

Imposter syndrome

Imposter syndrome is extremely common, even among successful, famous and talented people. Studies have found that imposter syndrome will affect 70% of all people at one time or another.[20] On your journey as an entrepreneur, you'll regularly be required to step out of your comfort zone. On the one hand, this is fantastic as you're given the opportunity to continually grow. On the other hand, it's the ideal conditions for imposter syndrome to strike. It can happen to any of us, at any age, regardless of our level of knowledge and expertise. It's also known as the imposter phenomenon, fraud syndrome and imposter experience. If you're experiencing imposter syndrome, then for no practical reason you may feel like a fraud or that your accomplishments came about as a result of luck, rather than your ability and hard work. Some of the signs and symptoms of imposter syndrome include:

- Self-doubt

- Attributing your success to external factors

- Sabotaging your own success

- Over-achieving

- Working harder than necessary

- Setting unrealistic goals

- Fear you won't live up to expectations

- Anxiety

Imposter syndrome is regularly triggered by a new experience such as setting up a new business, winning a new contract or public speaking in front of a new audience. Cultural expectations and what you perceive as society's definition of success can be another cause. Family expectations, comparison and perfectionism can also be a trigger. Perhaps you're already aware that imposter syndrome is something that you have experienced. If you're unsure, then answer these questions:

1. Do you worry and ruminate over minor errors in your work?

2. Do you attribute your success to luck?

3. Are you extremely sensitive to constructive criticism?

4. Do you feel like you will be 'found out' ultimately?

5. Do you downplay your success or expertise?

If you have answered yes to one or more of these questions and recognise some of the signs and symptoms listed, then it's important to identify ways to tackle imposter syndrome when it strikes. Remember, you're not alone. Some of the most successful people, including theoretical physicist Albert Einstein and civil rights activist Maya Angelou, have been identified as experiencing imposter syndrome.[21] Einstein is widely believed to have said, 'The exaggerated esteem in which my life work is held makes me very ill at ease. I feel compelled to think of myself as an involuntary swindler.'[22]

His imposter syndrome led to him fearing that he would ultimately be found a fraud, leaving him with doubts over his significant accomplishments, rather than seeing the high regard in which he was held as an extraordinary genius.

FOLLOW-UP WITH ALICE

Imposter syndrome is a massive part of her entrepreneurial journey and regularly experienced when thrown out of her comfort zone, but she has found that by identifying when imposter syndrome occurs, a simple change in her thought process can help her to grow. For example, public speaking is a trigger that Alice identified, but instead of accepting the thoughts telling her that she can't do it, Alice challenges and reframes them into a much more positive and productive light, for example, 'This is me stretching.'

The five core types of imposter syndrome

Dr Valerie Young has developed five core types of imposter syndrome: the perfectionist, the superhero, the expert, the natural genius and the soloist. Each named after the ways in which imposter syndrome presents itself, they have their own set of challenges.[23]

The perfectionist

The perfectionist sets goals for themselves that are excessively high, often to a point where the goal is unachievable. When the goal is not reached, the perfectionist will be hard on themselves. Rather than focusing on their achievements and strengths, the perfectionist will obsess over their flaws and the smallest mistakes. Often accused of being microman-agers, perfectionists find it hard to delegate and let go, worrying that their work will not be at a suitably high standard.

If you can relate to the perfectionist, then it's important to learn to take mistakes in your stride and remember that this is often how we learn and grow. Be mindful of the goals you are setting for yourself, stay ambitious but realistic and reward yourself for your accom-plishments. Practise delegating and letting go until this becomes more comfortable and you can learn to have faith in those around you.

The superhero

The superhero is often the last person to leave the office and finds downtime wasteful. They sacrifice personal interests for work, but this hard work is a coverup for insecurities. This feeling of inadequacy and the need to prove themselves can affect relationships with those around them and lead to physical and mental illness and burnout.

If you can relate to the superhero, then it's important to work on your own internal validation. Start nurturing your inner confidence by believing in your ability, recognising your accomplishments and responding to challenges in a constructive way. Recognise when you have done all that you can do and then learn to switch off and recharge.

The expert

The expert regularly feels that they need to improve their skills to succeed. Although continuous learning is important, the expert will often take this too far, booking on to courses more often than most as a way to justify their competence. Even though they are often highly knowledgeable and skilled, they fear being found out as a fraud and may shudder at the thought of being an expert.

If you can relate to the expert, then begin by recognising your achievements and accomplishments to date. The next time you consider booking on to a new course, question if you really need it and try asking those that support you what they think, too.

The natural genius

The natural genius has often excelled throughout their lives without too much effort. They judge their competence on ease and speed. They often set themselves excessively high goals, but when faced with a setback (such as not reaching these goals), their confidence is knocked. Worried they may not achieve something on the first try, they may avoid some challenges and feel uncomfortable participating in activities they don't feel good at.

If you can relate to the natural genius, then it's important to remember that we are all a work in progress. Be kind to yourself, step out of your comfort zone and embrace new challenges. Who knows what exciting things could develop as a result...

The soloist

The soloist tends to feel that they must accomplish tasks on their own to prove their worth. In their eyes, asking for help is a sign of weakness or incompetence, so they prefer to work on their own and demonstrate their own achievements.

If you can relate to the soloist, then it's important to start making a conscious effort to develop your skills in teamwork. The ability to work independently is essential, especially if you're running a business, but recognising the strength and achievements of the wider team can enhance your working relationships and your work output, too.

Overcoming imposter syndrome

If you can relate to one or more of the five types of imposter syndrome, then I hope you find the tips associated with each one useful. Over the next few weeks and months, try and be conscious of when imposter syndrome occurs. Follow these steps to become best placed to challenge this as you move forward on your entrepreneurial journey:

1. Recognise unhealthy patterns.

2. Build a network of like-minded, supportive people.

3. Recognise your accomplishments. Keep a file on your desk or on your laptop and fill it with your achievements. This could include certificates, thank you notes from

colleagues or customers, photos and reflections from your journey in business.

4. Stop comparing yourself to others. Remember, we are all on our own journey.

5. Find a mentor who has followed a similar path. They should offer reassurance when needed as someone who's, 'Been there, done that and worn the t-shirt.'

6. Address your inner critic.

7. Don't be afraid to reach out and ask for support. Most people are happy to help.

8. Refuse to let it hold you back.

Summary

Having resolve is an essential attribute for an entrepreneur when aiming to avoid burnout. Knowing how to deal with being overwhelmed by competing pressures, fixing the issues that make you procrastinate and facing off the dreaded imposter syndrome can all build a stronger 'you' when you need to focus on achieving your goals. Using the tools above will assist you in maintaining a relaxed, focused and confident approach to your work and dither, delay and self-doubt will no longer hold you back from realising your dreams and ambitions. As we conclude with this chapter, consider the following:

- Can you relate to feelings of overwhelm? How can you address these feelings?

- Will you make changes to prevent procrastination?

- What techniques will you put in place to overcome imposter syndrome?

FIVE
Opinion

A t some level, every choice made has a positive or negative consequence. Making value-based decisions gives you clarity and removes much of the stress and pressure around choosing the correct path. Being authentic allows your thoughts and actions to reflect what you truly believe, giving a much greater sense of wellbeing. This chapter about **opinion** in the PROSPER model will help you to define your values, make value-based decisions and explore the importance of authenticity.

Defining values

Values are important as they represent what we as individuals stand for. Our values, sometimes known as core beliefs, guide our thoughts, words and actions and can be seen as our internal navigation system. Our values help shape our future and are generally aligned with our purpose. By consistently honouring your personal values, you can experience fulfilment that is congruent to your true nature. In contrast, not honouring your personal values can lead to bad habits, a loss of integrity and decisions that aren't right for you and your life journey. Your core values can influence your relationships, how you show up at work and how to treat yourself.

CASE STUDY: RACHAEL

Before setting up her Safeguarding consultancy firm, Rachael was interviewed for a job within the NHS. The role was highly paid, with a great title and a range of other perks. During the interview, Rachael was told that the role would be 70% data lead. She explained that she didn't feel the role would be right for her. Although she doesn't mind looking at data, her passion and strengths lie in working with people. From earlier self-reflection work, she knew that working with numbers would get her stressed and make her feel uncomfortable. After the interview, Rachael was thanked for giving such an honest and authentic interview and encouraged to apply for any upcoming roles that may be more aligned. By firmly holding on to her values, Rachael was able to make a decision aligned with her authentic self and ultimately avoided putting herself in a position that would have made her unhappy, unproductive and potentially unhealthy.

Value-based decision-making

How many poor decisions have you made under pressure or in times of stress? As an entrepreneur, you will be required to make countless decisions every single day, which can become exhausting. Some of these are more important than others and some, if you don't get right, could have serious implications for your business. Imagine the impact of employing the wrong person for a role in your company or agreeing to a deal with the wrong investor. These high-pressure decisions require a clear and focused mind. Poor decision-making can also run into your personal life. Choices around relationships and friendships, financial commitments and daily lifestyle choices can all make an impact on your overall quality of life if not chosen correctly.

If you can relate to this, then you're not alone. As someone who has spent the majority of their adult life running at least one business, I have first-hand experience of how high levels of stress can impact on decisions, both personally and professionally. I have, however, learned that to avoid this, I must first take a step back to pause and reflect, particularly during times of heightened pressure. I believe that being mindful of your personal values and the values of your business will help provide a level of clarity, particularly when it's difficult to know where to turn for guidance or when your judgement feels clouded.

In the decision-making process, it's important to remember the level of intelligence our bodies provide us with. How often do you check in with how your body feels when you come to make a decision? Have you experienced 'butterflies' or a 'gut-wrenching' feeling? 'Trust your gut' is a well-used phrase, with science backing up the reason why. The gastrointestinal tract (also known as the gut) is sensitive to a range of emotions such as anxiety, excitement, anger, happiness and sadness. When you feel one of these emotions your gut is triggered and so you feel the response in your stomach. Interestingly, the connection between the gut and the brain goes both ways: a troubled intestine can also send signals to the brain. In times of high stress or anxiety, it may become difficult to tune into your gut instinct, so reaffirming value-based decisions is an essential skill to helping you stay on track.

You may already have a good indication of your values, or perhaps it's not something you have managed to reflect on before. The next, simple exercise can help you determine your values or check if they've changed. By carrying out this exercise, you can check that your personal and professional goals are aligned to your values as well as utilising this knowledge for future decision-making.

TASK: Determining your values

This exercise should take around fifteen minutes to complete. On a piece of paper, write down every value that resonates with you from the columns below. Try not to overthink your chosen words. If any others come to mind that aren't on the list, write those down, too.

Accuracy	Energy
Ambition	Enjoyment
Assertiveness	Equality
Attentive	Ethical
Authenticity	Excellence
Balance	Faith
Boldness	Fearless
Bravery	Freedom
Calm	Friendship
Capable	Fun
Community	Generosity
Compassion	Gratitude
Confidence	Greatness
Control	Growth
Courage	Health
Creativity	Honesty
Credibility	Hope
Decisive	Humility
Detailed	Humour
Dignity	Imagination
Efficiency	Independence
Empathy	Individuality

Inspiring

Integrity

Intelligence

Intuitive

Joy

Kindness

Knowledge

Leadership

Meaning

Motivation

Optimism

Originality

Passion

Patience

Persistence

Productivity

Purpose

Quality

Respect

Rigour

Security

Selfless

Simplicity

Stability

Standards

Success

Support

Thorough

Traditional

Transparency

Trust

Understanding

Uniqueness

Unity

Wisdom

The next step is to group the words together in a way that makes sense to you. Create a maximum of five groups. For example, several words may fall under 'happiness' or 'balance'.

Choose one word within each group that represents the entire group.

You can then create an actionable core value by adding a verb such as 'maintain, aid, prioritise, demonstrate, establish, implement, build'. For example, 'build resilience' and 'prioritise growth'.

Now that you have your core values, list them in order of priority. Place them somewhere that you can come back to for easy reference whenever you're faced with the need for an authentic decision.

Authenticity

How we express ourselves both reflects and affects who we are. A fear of authenticity stems from the fear of rejection. We've all had experiences in life that shape who we are. What we perceive as negative experiences and how they will be viewed by others may make us afraid of being authentic.

Being authentic allows your thoughts and actions to reflect what you truly believe, giving a much greater sense of wellbeing. Psychologists explain that in the process of healing, as an individual becomes more authentic, they become happier and their psychological wellbeing increases.[24] Acknowledging the real you by 'removing the mask' and embracing this can feel uncomfortable and even leave you feeling vulnerable, but to allow yourself to be authentic, you must be fully seen, removing perfectionism and the need to please others. Courage is where authenticity begins, by breaking down the walls you have built – not only with the people you feel comfortable with, but everyone you meet.

Friedrich Nietzsche was a German philosopher and precursor of existentialism, a cultural movement which considers freedom as the core of human existence. Nietzsche talked about the importance of living an authentic life. In existentialism, authenticity is the degree in which an individual's actions are in line with their beliefs and desires, despite pressure from society to behave in a particular manner. Nietzsche emphasised having the courage to be authentic and fight back against common beliefs. Taken from his philosophy, here are seven ways in which you can live a more authentic life:[25]

1. **Accept yourself as a totality:** Accept the person that you are by taking all

of your behaviour, your strengths and your weaknesses into account. Accept the things that you aren't great at and find ways to solve problems while still remaining authentic to who you are.

2. **Follow your own path:** Nietzsche explained that the path to self-discovery is a challenging one, but you must have the courage to overcome challenges that may lie ahead and listen to your inner voice to find your true calling rather than imitating others. Embrace your individual journey.

3. **Accept that you are different:** It was Nietzsche's belief that there is no right way to live your life. We should not judge the actions or beliefs of other people, and in the same way, we should also expect not to be judged by others. Choose to live your authentic life, even if it isn't popular or what society expects.

4. **Obey only yourself:** Nietzsche described two types of morality: master morality (which includes power and pride) and slave morality (which includes kindness and empathy). It was Nietzsche's belief that slave morality can make you too empathetic towards those that will take

advantage. Putting their needs and desires before your own can prevent you from acting in an authentic way. Instead, balance empathy with self-confidence and self-respect. For example, if you feel someone is taking advantage of your good nature and you're having to do things that you don't want to, then have the courage to speak up to them and don't allow yourself to be controlled by their requests.

5. **Don't be ashamed:** Nietzsche explained that feeling ashamed can prevent us from being our authentic selves through the fear of further embarrassment or shame. Someone in this position can be easily controlled by individuals using shame to keep them in their place. If you've made a mistake, learn from it and remember that it does not define you. When you no longer accept shame, you can live authentically and freely.

6. **Forgive yourself:** Remember that as humans, we make mistakes. Be kind to your younger self – you didn't know then what you know now. Learn to forgive yourself for past mistakes.

7. **Live dangerously:** At all costs, preserve the authenticity of who you are. In the words of Nietzsche, 'That which does not kill me, makes me stronger.'[26]

FOLLOW-UP WITH RACHAEL

Authenticity is Rachael's most important value. 'Being authentic to myself has allowed me to be happy in my own skin, my own thoughts, to own my personality and to also choose my own path in life rather than accept limiting beliefs and to go with perceived norms and expectations,' she says. 'It has not only shaped my career and allowed me to excel in what I love, but to also refuse the things that bring me discomfort.'

Other values that Rachael holds close to her include honesty, integrity and empathy. 'Again, I think they just add to being authentic and allow me to be the best version of myself to help others, which, in essence, is exactly what I do. I am happier, healthier and much more productive in every aspect of my life since figuring out my values and how they help me connect to people and also render better service for customers.'

Being authentic in a filtered world

It can be easy to forget that social media profiles are often just highlights of our real lives.

With so many filtered and significant elements of our daily reality removed, social media can influence its users to believe that showing the best version of themselves is the best way to get validation, through likes and follows from others. Social media now plays a vital part both in how we express ourselves and what we observe around us. A recent report revealed that in 2022, the worldwide average daily social media usage amounted to 147 minutes per day,[27] so it's important that we understand the potential implications on our mental health and wellbeing and how we can maintain authenticity. There are three factors that can assist with this:

1. **Self-esteem:** It's important to remember not to believe everything you see on social media. Digitally manipulated photos can be created in a matter of seconds through apps that can change facial features and even body shape. It's a worrying trend, particularly for younger generations growing up with unrealistic perceptions of body image. Creating a false perception, whether it's in lifestyle, success or physical appearance, can cause lower self-esteem for those observing, as well as the

individual not truly investing in their own authenticity.

2. **Negative posts:** Negativity in any situation can be problematic. To build resilience, it is essential that you are able to feel positive and show gratitude. If you're logging into your social media account to read through negative posts that don't make you feel good, then make a change to stop this. Unfollowing or blocking an account may seem drastic, but if you're serious about improving your wellbeing then having a digital spring-clean is a great way to get started. Being authentic will attract like-minded followers and you may feel less inclined to follow people or organisations that don't resonate with your values or beliefs.

3. **Social interaction:** I've personally used LinkedIn as a way of connecting with new business contacts and have had a positive response, but picking up the phone or meeting in person is still key to building strong relationships. Although it's been reported that social media has changed the way we interact with one another, it's often for convenience rather than quality and we can develop superficial relationships. A top

tip from social media experts is to be clear on what purpose you would like social media to serve for you and only be present on platforms that meet these requirements. It's essential to consider the type of social interactions you require, the time you want to commit and the type of content you would like to share.

Summary

Having defined and well-structured opinions is vital as an entrepreneur. You have to be decisive and, at times, make decisions at breakneck speed. The best way to do this is to stay authentic and true to your values when casting your opinions. Repeatedly identifying your core values in the exercises above will help you focus your mind on who you are, what you are about and what you stand for. This will help you to remain authentic. As we come to the end of this chapter, take a few moments to consider the following:

- What are your values and have they changed over time?

- Are there ways in which you can live more authentically?

SIX

Strength Of Body And Mind

A healthy mind and body are essential for everyday living, but they are also something that we must nurture, like an Olympic athlete or astronaut would be required to do to achieve optimal performance. This section of the PROSPER model provides insight into a wide range of techniques to help keep your mind and body healthy, including sleep, exercise, the importance of getting outdoors, mindfulness, gratitude and positivity and giving back to support **strength** of mind and body.

Sleep

The importance of sleep on health

It's well documented that we should aim to get around eight hours of sleep per night.[28] Most adults will need this amount of sleep to fully rest and rejuvenate, but there are a few individuals that can manage with much less. Often when you can't sleep, the thought of feeling tired the next day causes increased anxiety. It then becomes much more difficult to relax and you may find yourself 'clock watching' – I'm sure we've all been there. If you find yourself in this situation, try to relax. The occasional poor night's sleep will leave you feeling tired the next day, but it won't affect your health. However, continuous sleepless nights can make it difficult to concentrate and make decisions. You may feel tired all of the time, which can affect your mental health and wellbeing. A lack of sleep can also affect physical health and has been linked to high blood pressure, diabetes and being overweight.

Sleep cycles

Parallel to the duration of sleep time we require is sleep quality, ensuring that the time spent sleeping is in fact restorative. This involves consistently and smoothly moving through each sleep stage in the cycle.

Stage one normally lasts up to five minutes as you start to fall asleep. Activity in the body and brain start to slow down and, if undisturbed, the body will move on to stage two. At this stage, the body enters a more subdued state. Eye movement stops, temperature drops, breathing slows down and muscles become more relaxed. This stage can last around ten to twenty-five minutes and increase with each cycle. As you move into stage three, you enter a deep sleep and the body relaxes even further. Studies have shown that this stage is critical for bodily recovery and growth. Evidence has also shown that deep sleep contributes to memory and creativity. Lasting around twenty to forty minutes, deep sleep generally gets shorter with each cycle. The final stage is REM, which commonly starts around ninety minutes into your sleep cycle. This sleep stage is believed to be essential to a range of cognitive functions, including memory and learning. REM sleep is probably best known for vivid dreaming, which could be a result of the increased brain activity during this stage. Within your first sleep cycle, REM only lasts a few minutes, but this tends to build with each cycle.[29]

Each sleep stage is important in supporting brain and body recuperation and development. People with apnoea can be frequently awoken during earlier stages, missing out on vital deep sleep and REM, while individuals with insomnia may struggle to get enough total sleep to meet the time needed in each stage, impacting on physical, emotional and mental health.

Improving sleep

There are a number of ways in which the quality of your sleep can be improved to help you wake each morning feeling fully rested. To begin, first assess the reasons why your sleep is being affected:

- Consider the temperature of the room and the light and noise levels.

- How comfortable is your bed?

- Do you look forward to relaxing in bed each evening?

- At what time do you have your last meal?

- Could you be eating too late or going to bed hungry?

- When was your last caffeinated drink?

- When do you switch off digital devices?

- Do you have a relaxing bedtime routine?

Once you have identified some of the key issues, you can start to make changes to your evening routine. By watching TV or flicking through social media, you can unintentionally evoke a range of emotions that aren't helpful for sleep, such as anger or anxiety. It's important that you wind down and relax ready for sleep, so be mindful of the activities that you're engaging in. How you do this will differ from person to person. Essential oils such as lavender and cedarwood, chamomile tea and a warm bath have been known to help aid sleep. If you find yourself ruminating over events that have happened or the things that you need to do, try writing them down. Getting these thoughts out of your mind and onto paper can help you to focus on activities that will help you to relax. (Read more about switching off in Chapter 8.)

A comfortable bed is essential. Choose cotton sheets which are breathable and help to prevent overheating. When choosing a mattress, make sure it provides enough support for your back, while not being so firm that your hips and shoulders are under pressure.

A constant lack of sleep can become a serious problem and affect your health, wellbeing and safety, particularly if you drive or are responsible for operating heavy machinery. If this is the case, then it's important that you speak to a medical professional who can provide additional support.

Exercise

Being physically active on a regular basis is one of the most important things you can do for your overall health and quality of life. Physical activity can help manage weight and reduce your risk of serious illnesses and diseases, including Type 2 diabetes, cardiovascular disease, dementia, depression, anxiety and many types of cancer. Regular physical activity can also strengthen muscles and bones, and improve cognitive function and physical fitness. Exercise is well known for releasing endorphins and even on the days that you don't feel like exercising, you'll be pumped up with feel-good hormones and ready to tackle whatever lies ahead by the end of your workout.

Although physical activity is essential for health and preventing early death, the British Heart Foundation revealed that 38% of adults in the UK do not meet the physical activity recommendations.[30] Key reasons for low activity levels include lack of time, low energy levels, poor drive and determination, fear of injury, few options and little support.

Recommended physical activity guidelines

The recommended physical activity guidelines are to do at least 150 minutes of moderate intensity activity per week. Moderate intensity activity should raise your heart rate, make your breath faster and make you feel warm. Examples include cycling, walking briskly, water aerobics and mowing the lawn. If you're struggling to fit physical activity into your weekly routine, then break these 150 minutes up into manageable chunks that work around your schedule. For example, if you have more free time on a weekend, you could do 60 minutes of activity on a Saturday and 60 minutes of activity on a Sunday, leaving just 30 minutes to spread out across the rest of the week – that's just 6 minutes Monday to Friday.

If you're physically fit and prefer higher intensity exercise, then just 75 minutes of activity will help you see the same benefits as 150 minutes of moderate activity. High intensity exercise will leave you feeling out of breath. It includes running, swimming, aerobics and sports such as football and squash. Many moderate activities can become higher intensity by increasing your effort.

On two days per week, you should also aim to do muscle strengthening exercises using all of the major muscle groups. Attending the gym to lift weights or joining a class such as yoga, Pilates or body-tone that incorporates weight-bearing exercises will help you to achieve this goal. There may be activities that you perform regularly that will also contribute, such as lifting heavy shopping bags, manual labour and carrying children. The key to increasing physical activity levels is to make it consistent and manageable.[31]

At the office

There are many ways you can increase your physical activity levels while at work. Some examples include taking the stairs as much as possible, walking around while you're on the phone and stretching for a couple of minutes during your break. Implementing these small changes daily will increase your overall weekly step count and activity levels. I particularly enjoy a walking meeting and find that walking in the sunshine with endorphins pumping helps boost creativity. Alternatively, why not use your break time to walk with colleagues. Using this time to properly switch off by enjoying the fresh air, noticing your surroundings and keeping your focus in the present moment can help you to return to the office feeling refreshed and energised. Consider your home, office and social life to see where small, manageable changes can be made.

At home

There are lots of simple ways that can help you become more active around the home. Consider the activities that involve you being most sedentary, for example watching television. To combat this sedentary activity, each time the TV adverts appear, make a conscious effort to get up and move around the house, or at the start of each programme use the first ten to twenty minutes to carry out some mobilising exercises and stretches.

Have you considered how cleaning and gardening can help increase your physical activity levels? By increasing the intensity, you'll also be increasing the level of impact. Not only are you reaping the benefits of physical activity, but tackling the household chores too: a win/win situation. If you have stairs at home, then make an effort to go up and down regularly. In fact, the stairs don't limit you to only 'up and down' exercises – your bottom stair can be used to perform exercises such as raised push-ups, dips and lunges. Lots of people get their steps in walking the dog each day. If you're a dog owner, shake up your routine by trying a new, longer route or find a social dog walking club where you can discover new walks while enjoying some social interaction.

Friends and family

Physical activity shouldn't feel like a chore. The more fun you have, the more likely you are to keep it up. Sharing the experience of a dance or fitness class with a friend or family member can be great fun. Attending a class with someone else also keeps you more accountable, as you don't want to let the other person down. Bike rides, football, netball and dodgeball might be something that you haven't participated in since you were a child, but these activities can be enjoyed by everyone. Get your friends or family involved – it might even bring out your competitive streak.

Getting outdoors

If you're anything like me, then you'll already appreciate the impact that taking a walk in nature can have on clearing the mind and providing an injection of feel-good hormones. Just being in nature, whether that's along the coastline, at a local park or in the countryside, has the ability to boost mood and improve vitality. Research has shown that exposure to nature can reduce high blood pressure, respiratory tract illness and cardiovascular illness. It has been recorded that 'feeling part of nature has been shown to significantly correlate with life satisfaction, vitality, meaningfulness, happiness and lower cognitive anxiety.'[32]

There has also been significant evidence demonstrating the benefits of sunlight on health and wellbeing. Vitamin D, also known as the sunshine vitamin, is absorbed through the skin from sunlight. Regular sun exposure is the most natural way to get enough vitamin D. It helps the body absorb calcium and phosphate from our diet. This prevents our bones from becoming weak and soft which can lead to breakages and deformities. A recent study also found that post-surgery exposure to sunlight decreased stress and pain, minimising the need for painkillers by 21%.[33] It is believed that sunlight increases beta-endorphins in the skin, resulting in pain-killing effects. More commonly known is that sunlight increases serotonin levels, which makes you happy. Low levels of serotonin are associated with a higher risk of seasonal affective disorder. This is a form of depression often triggered by the changing seasons when levels of sunlight are reduced.

Research suggests that you should aim to get between ten and thirty minutes of sunlight several times per week.[34] Exposure time will vary depending on how sensitive your skin is to sunlight. For example, people with darker skin may require more exposure time than those with fair skin who burn quickly. As the long summer days draw to a close, you may find yourself leaving for work and returning home in the dark and wintry weather. The reduced daylight hours can make it increasingly challenging to get enough sun exposure outside of your working hours. Going outside, even on a cloudy, rainy day, can still provide mood-lifting and immunity-boosting vitamin D, so make the most of those break times and get outdoors as much as you can. In the UK, the NHS recommends that during autumn and winter, everyone should consider taking a daily vitamin D supplement.[35] Foods including oily fish, egg yolks and mushrooms all contain vitamin D, but getting enough vitamin D from your diet alone can be difficult.

If spending more time outdoors is something that you'd like to achieve, then consider scheduling this time into your weekly calendar. You could try walking instead of driving or taking public transport where possible. Don't wait for the perfect day – as the saying goes, 'There's no such thing as bad weather, just unsuitable clothing.' Get those waterproofs on, wrap up warm and start exploring.

Mindfulness

Mindfulness is the practice of purposefully and non-judgementally paying attention to what's happening to you in a particular moment in time. Instead of living life on autopilot, mindfulness allows you to be completely aware of what's going on around you. Research has shown that the benefits of this include an increased ability to relax, which helps to manage stress and reduce anxiety. Studies have also found a link between mindfulness practice and brain activity that supports memory, learning and emotions.[36] As you become more mindful, it's likely that you'll become more aware of how often your mind is racing, as well as when your focus shifts from the present moment to the past or the future.

Mindfulness can easily be practised throughout the day by simply choosing a moment in which to be present rather than letting your thoughts race. Try the next two exercises to get started.

TASK: Mindful eating

This a great way to implement mindfulness practice into your everyday life. It can also help you to recognise when you're full and avoid overeating.

To begin, remove any distraction such as your mobile phone and turn off the TV if it's in the room. Keep your focus on your food, chewing slowly and savouring each bite. Pay attention to the aroma of the food, its texture and flavours.

Once complete, reflect on what a difference being present made to how you felt before the meal and how it made you feel about the food you ate.

TASK: Five senses

This exercise can be completed in just five minutes during your break or outside of your working day. Spend one minute focusing on each of the five senses.

To begin, sit in a comfortable, upright position with your feet flat on the floor and your arms in a relaxed position. Take a deep breath in and exhale fully. Continue to breathe deeply throughout the exercise, keeping your focus on the present moment.

- First, notice what you can see around you, including colours, patterns, shapes and textures. What colour do you see most? Are there textures that you haven't noticed before?

- What can you hear? Can you hear your breathing or any sounds in the distance? Are there any subtle sounds that may have gone unnoticed? Close your eyes if this helps.

- Pick up on the smells in the environment around you. Is someone cooking? Are smells entering the room from an open window? What subtle scents can you pick up?

- Identify what you can taste. Focus on the taste in your mouth as you breathe or run your tongue over your teeth. Alternatively, if you have a snack or a drink with you, then use this time to notice all of its flavours.

- Finally, notice the texture of where your hands are placed. Feel the pressure of your feet against the floor, noticing any textures beneath them. Feel the different textures of any other objects close by.

Gently bring all of your senses back and take a moment to compare how you're feeling now compared to when you began the exercise.

Gratitude and positivity

Gratitude helps shift your focus from what you feel is missing in your life, to appreciating what is already present. Psychologists Michael

McCullough of Southern Methodist University and Robert Emmons of the University of California carried out an experiment on gratitude and its impact on wellbeing. In the study, hundreds of people were split into three groups and asked to write about their daily experiences. Group one wrote down things they were grateful for that day, such as family and waking up on a morning. Group two wrote down things that had bothered them, such as finances depleting fast and a friend not appreciating a kind gesture. Group three wrote about any experiences from the day. The results of the study indicated that practising daily gratitude resulted in greater energy, optimism and life satisfaction. The group that practised gratitude were also 25% happier than those that had not.[37]

When you practise gratitude regularly, you tap into neuroplasticity, which strengthens positive new brain cell connections. The power of positive thinking has been shown to have many physical and mental benefits. A positive mindset can give you more confidence, improve your mood and even reduce the likelihood of developing conditions such as hypertension, depression and other stress-related disorders.

All this sounds great, but what does the 'power of positive thinking' really mean? Positive thinking can come in the form of positive imagery, positive self-talk or optimism. If you want to be effective in being positive, you'll need to start implementing a number of simple, but effective methods into your daily routine. Read through these suggestions to see which you could start practising today:

- **Start the day with a positive affirmation:** How you start the morning sets the tone for the rest of the day. Have you ever woken up late and then felt like nothing good happened the rest of the day? It is likely this is because you started the day with a pessimistic view that carried into other events. Instead of letting this happen, start the day with a positive affirmation. Talk to yourself with statements like, 'Today will be a good day,' or, 'I'm going to do well today.' You'll be amazed at how much your day improves.

- **Focus on the good things:** You're probably going to encounter obstacles throughout your day. When you encounter challenges, try and focus on the benefits, no matter how small they seem. For example, if you're stuck in traffic, think about how you now have time to listen to the rest of your favourite playlist. If the shop is out of the food you wanted for dinner, think about the benefit of trying something new.

- **Find humour in challenging situations:** Allow yourself to experience humour in even the most trying situations. Remind yourself that this situation will probably make for a good story later and try to crack a joke about it.

- **Turn failures into lessons:** We all make mistakes and experience failure in different ways. Instead of focusing on how you failed, try and focus on what you're going to do differently next time and turn your failure into a lesson.

- **Change negative self-talk into positive self-talk:** Negative self-talk is often hard to notice. You might think, 'I'm so bad at this,' or, 'I shouldn't have tried that.' Recognise that these thoughts turn into feelings and can impact your perceptions of yourself. When you catch yourself doing this, stop and replace those negative messages with positive ones. For example, 'I'm so bad at this,' could become, 'Once

I get more practice, I'll be way better at this.'

- **Focus on the present:** Not today, not this hour, only this exact moment. You might be getting stressed, but what in this exact moment is happening that's so bad? Forget the incident or comment that made you stressed five minutes ago. Forget what might happen five minutes from now. Focus on this one, individual moment. In most situations, you'll find it's not as bad as you imagined. Most sources of negativity stem from a memory or the imagination of the future. Stay in the present moment.

Giving back

If 'giving back' is something that you already regularly do, then you'll have experienced first-hand the benefits in doing so. Backed by research, acts of giving and kindness can help combat stress and anxiety, provide a sense of purpose or reward, improve self-confidence and build connections with others.[38]

CASE STUDY: BILL

Dr Bill Scott OBE is the chief executive of the Teesside engineering company, Wilton Universal Group. Wilton was declared the fastest growing company in the North-East of England in 2010 and 2011.

Bill had already taken calls from three people in need of his help, advice and support on the day of our interview. It typifies what he is about. He feels lucky to be in a position to give something back to others and says, 'Everything you give back, you have ten times coming back to you.' A philanthropist, Bill supports a range of charities and community groups offering mentoring to local entrepreneurs in his spare time, providing invaluable advice, guidance and support. A great listener, you can tell just from talking to him that he has a wealth of experience, a desire to help and plenty of empathy. His positivity is contagious. Indeed, he says, 'In my world, my cup is always overflowing, never half full.' Little wonder then that the people he supports ultimately act upon his advice, creating a community of individuals who give something back to society.

Ways of giving back

- Ask friends, family and colleagues how they are and take the time to really listen to their answers.

- Spend time with friends, relatives or neighbours who need support or may be feeling isolated.

- Offer to help someone you know with tasks they may find challenging such as cutting the lawn or picking up some shopping.

- Volunteer in your local community at a charity or social enterprise.

Scottish author and government reformer Samuel Smiles said, 'Good actions give strength to ourselves and inspire good action in others.'[39] When you lead a busy life, it can be hard to find time to do anything outside of your weekly routine, but if you can spare even just a small amount of time, the benefits of volunteering are enormous. Not only does volunteering offer vital support for worthwhile causes, but as previously mentioned, the benefits can be significant to you too, helping to improve your health and happiness:

- **It connects you to others:** For those who are less outgoing than others, it gives you the opportunity to develop your social skills and to build relationships with people who share your interests. Not only is this good for building professional relationships, but also for making friends.

- **It can help reduce stress, anger and anxiety:** Nothing relieves stress better than a meaningful connection to another person or people. Working with animals has also been shown to improve mood and reduce stress and anxiety.

- **It can help you stay physically healthy:** As discussed above, physical activity is one of the most important things you can do for your overall health and quality of life. Physical activity can help manage weight and reduce your risk of serious illnesses and diseases. By volunteering in a role that keeps you active, you can reap the benefits of regular exercise.

- **It can increase self-confidence:** Volunteering and doing good for others can provide a natural sense of accomplishment. The better you feel about yourself, the more likely you are to have a positive view of your life.

- **It can advance your career, or in the case of a business owner, your own company:** For example, if you're considering setting up a business in a new market, it can help you get experience in your area of interest and meet people in the field. It also helps you acquire useful skills like teamwork, communication, problem-solving and project planning. Many volunteering opportunities provide extensive training. For example, you may become experienced in fundraising or gain extensive knowledge of history while volunteering in a museum.

- **It's a fun and easy way to explore your interests and passions:** It can be meaningful and interesting, not to mention a timely and energising escape from your daily routine. Many people volunteer in fields which overlap with their hobbies. For example, if you have a desk job, but wish to spend more time outdoors, you may volunteer at a community garden or walk dogs for an animal shelter.

CASE STUDY: SOPHIE

Multi-award-winning businesswoman and proud mum, Sophie enjoys supporting and promoting the North-East of England. She is a supporter of Northern Power Women, co-founder of City Ladies Networking and the voluntary Chair of Smart Works, Newcastle. She explains how rewarding volunteering in her role at Smart Works has been. 'I had told my team at the time that I was saying no to anything beyond my current roles for a while, except if Smart Works came up as an opportunity. A few weeks later, the Chair role was advertised. I think it resonates as I have a background in employability and a passion for supporting women. The Chair role was the icing on the cake, as it is a position of influence, which builds on my skillset,' she says. 'I always feel happy when spending a day on Smart Works activity and it lifts my mood.'

Summary

Staying physically active and getting adequate amounts of sleep can be the difference between feeling tired and unmotivated to feeling refreshed and raring to go. You can set yourself goals and build specific times for exercising into your routine, as well as impromptu activities within the workplace or at home, incorporating the great outdoors where you can. Your sleep is critical and should be a priority. Try some of the techniques detailed in this chapter and Chapter 8 to help you switch off from a busy day's work, relax and reboot as you drift into dreamland.

Keeping your mind healthy can be tough, especially when you have tight deadlines, challenging encounters and lots of personalities to juggle in your business life. Using techniques such as mindfulness, positivity and gratitude can provide a sense of calm and clarity when life can seem hectic or overwhelming. Take a moment now to:

- Consider which techniques you would like to use

- Commit to reflecting on the difference each has made at the end of each week

PART THREE
PHASE TWO OF THE PROSPER MODEL

In Part Three of this book, you will be guided through the final phase of the PROS-PER model (Productivity, Equilibrium and Reward). This section will help you discover ways to implement the techniques shared in Part Two into your daily routine. I will also share with you additional factors to consider to maintain health and wellbeing while achieving your ambitions at work and at home.

SEVEN

Productivity

There is no denying that wellbeing and **productivity** go hand in hand. This chapter will help you explore techniques to increase productivity, including ways to enhance your working environment, improve time management and develop a harmonious support network.

Work environment

The design of your workspace can play a significant role in your productivity and business success. How your environment makes you feel can influence your mood, motivation, creativity and interaction with others, so it's essential to consider how your workspace may be influencing your current performance and wellbeing. Making just a few small changes can make a significant difference:

- **Natural light:** As discussed in Chapter 6, the weather can play a significant role in how we feel, so it's unsurprising that the level of natural light in our workspace can have the same effect. Poor levels of natural light in your work environment can lead to problems such as headaches and eye strain, whereas a good level of natural light can help keep the brain alert as well as improve mood. Research has shown that carefully considered lighting can help improve productivity,[40] so if possible, work close to a window or under a skylight. If you're unable to do this, add light where you can and get outdoors during break times.

- **Indoor plants:** By bringing plants into your workspace, you can experience numerous health benefits. They oxygenate the air while removing pollutants and bacteria. Research has shown that plants also help increase humidity and moisture in the air. This can help prevent sore throats and irritated eyes as a result of dryness, particularly during the winter months when we turn on the heating.[41] Bringing plants indoors can offer similar benefits to being out in nature, such as helping to improve blood pressure, reducing anxiety and promoting feelings of vitality, which ultimately help improve productivity.

- **Pictures and prints:** Create an inspiring environment that can help you to stay motivated by adding pictures that help inspire you. This could be a picture of your favourite landscape or travel destination, past achievements or inspirational quotes. In my home office, I have all of these on display while sticking to a coordinated colour theme so that my walls don't feel too 'busy' or cluttered.

- **Aromatherapy:** I'm a big fan of aromatherapy and all of the benefits it brings. Smell is one of our strongest senses, with the ability to influence brain activity. An uplifting smell can not only change the feeling of your surroundings, but help you to be more productive. Add your favourite candle or diffuse essential oils to start seeing the benefits.

- **Music:** Can you list a handful of songs that help boost your mood? Perhaps there's a song that helps you to get motivated for the day ahead or a big event. Pop these in a playlist to help you feel more relaxed or productive throughout the working day, on your way into the office or on your journey home.

FOLLOW-UP WITH ALICE

Based on Alice's experience in interior design and as a successful entrepreneur, she highlights that calculating the amount of time you spend in your workspace provided ample justification for investing in it. It should be warm, comfortable and feel homely. If you are working from home, Alice advises that you choose your space carefully. For example, a lot of people will choose the smallest room in their home as their home office, but swapping this space for the spare room will provide more space for a range of seating and increased light. Making your workspace a pleasant place to be will improve how you feel working there and ultimately impact on your wellbeing and productivity, whether it's at home or at work.

Time management

Time is irreplaceable and one of the most important things we have. It's one of the few things that can't be bought and holds such a high value when spent doing the things we most enjoy and with the people we love. As a new mum, my time feels more precious than ever. Conscious of not wanting to waste precious time that could be spent with my baby boy, my focus each week is on my work priorities with little to no deviation. More focused than ever, staying assigned to these priorities and tackling the most essential tasks helps me to increase productivity while also allowing me the time to recharge. During my fourteen years in business, I have also found these techniques to useful:

- **Planning is key:** By regularly reviewing your diary, you can analyse if you're using your time as effectively as possible. Plot both work and leisure time into your diary and make a note when work overflows into leisure time. This will help you to make a thorough analysis at the end of each week of what has worked well and what needs improvement. Remember, your leisure time is just as important as your work time. Having a detailed schedule of your week ahead based on your current priorities can help increase productivity while also reducing stress and overwhelm. Depending on what works best for you, this could be a breakdown of tasks hour by hour, or just a bullet list of tasks for the day. Once your plan is in place, stick to it as much as possible and avoid unnecessary distractions – often easier said than done, but practising this discipline will help.

- **Delegate where possible:** As the founder of a business, you know it inside out, what works and what doesn't. You've worked hard to get to this point, building a brand and product or service that your clients value and trust. Letting go of elements of your work can feel like a challenge, but what are the potential results of not doing so? Perhaps your business growth is halted? You struggle to take downtime? Face the possibility of burnout? Recognising your strengths and weaknesses can help you to identify how a person with a differing skillset can create a stronger team for greater productivity. Successful entrepreneurs know that if you hire people that are better than you in their area of expertise and give them the work you don't have time for or you're unsure of, they are likely to do this much quicker than you can and even help you to learn in the process. Outsourcing and using freelance contractors could be another option to help free up your time for the things that only you can do.

- **Find automating solutions:** With the development of technology and the software as a service business model, it has never been easier to use apps and online services to automate and often streamline your business processes. From scheduling social media and generating invoices to keeping on track with a project and up to date with employee documentation, software can free up time as well as create efficiencies within the business.

- **Avoid multitasking:** How often do you find yourself multitasking throughout the day? It may feel like an efficient way to save time while getting as much done as possible, but research has shown that focusing on one task at a time is better for productivity and performance.[42] Giving yourself the time to fully focus on the task at hand – giving it the attention it deserves – can prevent careless mistakes that may need correcting later. It also saves time that would otherwise be wasted by continually turning your attention from one activity to another.

- **Take regular breaks:** When you're running low on time and feel like you have a million and one things to do then taking a break can feel counterproductive, but taking a short break to properly recharge can help increase focus once you return to your task. This improves productivity while also helping your wellbeing. A well-known technique for this is the Pomodoro technique developed by Francesco Cirillo in the late 1980s.[43]

TASK: Pomodoro technique

First, set a timer for twenty-five minutes. During this time, focus on a single task. Once the alarm goes off, take a five-minute break before starting your next task for a further twenty-five minutes. Repeat this process four times before taking a longer twenty to twenty-five-minute break. If the task you're aiming to complete is going to take a longer period of time, then break it down into smaller, manageable chunks.

I find the Pomodoro technique is a great way to stay focused and work on the current priorities for the day. Practising this technique also helps you to become more aware of the distractions around you which could be impacting on your daily level of productivity.

Support network

Research has shown that entrepreneurship can be a lonely journey. Isolation was cited as one of the biggest entrepreneurial challenges in the Self-Employment Review carried out by Julie Deane, founder of the Cambridge Satchel Company. Although the majority of self-employed entrepreneurs reported that they would not go back into employment, 25% stated that they missed having colleagues. The review highlights that, 'Understanding that there is no one else to work with, that it can be a solitary and often lonely occupation is one of the issues that people need to recognize comes with the territory.'[44]

Loneliness is closely linked to an individual's mental health. Studies have shown that individuals feeling lonely over a long period of time have an increased risk of a range of mental health problems such as anxiety, depression and low self-esteem.[45] Social well-being can be improved by building a network of authentic, supportive and like-minded individuals both in your work environment and in your personal life. Our relationships with others can give us a sense of belonging, and help us to feel valued and good about ourselves. They can help us to reduce stress and worry through the opportunity to share problems and seek support. They can also stimulate and inspire us through conversation and laughter.

CASE STUDY: SIMONE

Simone Roche MBE is the founder and CEO of Northern Power Women. A community of over 85,000 individuals, it is a catalyst for driving change while uniting businesses and individuals. It was on a train heading back to her hometown that Simone made the conscious decision to change the narrative of diversity within the north. She says, 'I had been working in and around gender equality for years, and on that train, it occurred that I was always up and down on the West Coast Main Line to London town where all the gender equality conversations where happening – I decided I'd change the geography of where the conversation was happening to the north.'

Simone launched a campaign for all voices to have their say on the future of the North. The campaign, which helped showcase role models, was a huge success and, 'The hashtag #Northernpowerwomen went bonkers!' she says. Simone believes this is partly due to a fantastic sense of northern pride and support for inclusivity. Since founding Northern Power Women, Simone has built a vast community from all genders, backgrounds and socio-economic groups across the north. 'We talk about the six degrees of separation. I think it's often just two. If you're connected with the right groups, or even subgroups, it's where that magic can happen,' she says. 'We set up WhatsApp groups to enable those easy exchanges. They create a safe space to check out an idea, ask for advice and share good news with others who will celebrate success.'

Two (or more) heads are often better than one when aiming to create big results. Bringing together a diverse group of individuals to collaborate on a common goal can increase the success of a project through the act of sharing expertise. As well as helping you to achieve more, collaboration can make problem-solving easier and can open up new opportunities.

It can be hard to decide which networks to be part of, and Simone suggests looking for like-minded people. 'If it's not for you, it doesn't mean it's not a great network or community, it's just not right for you at that moment in time.' Be curious, ask questions and consider why you want to be part of these networks. 'Identify what the purpose of those organisations are, for example a book club might involve coming together once a month after you've read a few chapters of a book. Is that something that you can, and would like to, commit to?' she says. Ask yourself how much time you've got to give and whether this a place for you or a place to give back. Don't be afraid to ask organisations what you get out of it. As Simone says, 'If you're going to give your time and bring your energy, then it's definitely a two-way street.'

Negative social interactions

As well as enhancing your social wellbeing through authentic, like-minded and supportive relationships with others, you must also address the impact of negative social interactions, recognise when these occur and implement effective techniques to protect your wellbeing. A negative interaction can be presented by someone being intrusive and showing poor boundaries. They may be overly critical, argumentative, constantly negative and unable to accept responsibility. If you find yourself in this situation and you must continue to deal with this person, then it's essential to protect your energy when negativity occurs and not allow their problems to become yours. Here are three ways to assist:

- **Be aware of those that drain your energy:** The term 'energy vampire' is often used for someone who leaves you feeling emotionally drained. Although not always obvious when you first meet them, trust your instinct with this. You may find yourself feeling irritable and negative, with a loss of energy. Physical signs can also include muscle tension and headaches that seem to develop when you're in their company.

- **Set firm limits:** It's sometimes the case that you can't detach completely from someone that may be having a negative effect on your social wellbeing, particularly in the case of family members or co-workers, so it's important to set firm limits. For example, for those that consume a lot of your time and energy, be clear on how much time you have available. At the end of that time period, politely disengage.

- **Call it out:** How often have you experienced unfavourable behaviour and chosen to either ignore it or complain about it to someone else? As both of these are natural reactions, it can be easy for this to become your 'go to' behaviour, but this can be counterproductive. It's often the case that negative behaviours are unintentional and without the intervention of someone else they can continue to go unnoticed. For example, someone making an insensitive comment might think they're making a joke. It's important to highlight what's really going on to educate and enact change. Calling out unfavourable behaviour when you see it can transform negative behaviours in a positive way.

Summary

Productivity is key to the success of any flourishing business. To be as productive as possible, you need to set the scene. This includes setting up your office or workspace in a way that makes your work easier, is relaxing and benefits your health. Make sure there's lots of natural light, plants dotted around the room and comfortable furniture. Manage your time as effectively as possible to help reduce stress and create a lifestyle that works for you. Finally, surround yourself with positive and supportive people, while also knowing when and how to deal with individuals having a negative effect. As we conclude with this chapter, consider the following:

- Do you feel inspired and productive in your workspace?

- Could your time be used more effectively?

- Who is in your support network?

EIGHT
Equilibrium

B alance means that your life will find its own **equilibrium** and ensure that when stressors and strains come along, they won't throw you off your direction. You'll be able to manage it and feel in control of your own destiny. In this section of the PROSPER model you will explore work-life balance and techniques to switch off and maintain harmony.

Work-life balance

Successfully achieving a healthy work-life balance can support greater achievement in the workplace, as well as improved wellbeing and happiness. In contrast, not achieving a healthy work-life balance can result in increased stress levels, exhaustion, illness and burnout. Although at times work-life balance may feel unattainable, it is possible to be successful in your professional career while also maintaining a healthy and fulfilling personal life. What this balance looks like will be different to everyone and is rarely in equal measure.

Research has found that major challenges contributing to poor work-life balance include unrealistic demands, unsupportive relationships and high levels of stress.[46] It has become almost normal behaviour for work to creep into our personal time. As a business owner, this will almost certainly be the case from time to time and it's essential to identify when this is to your detriment. Living in an 'always on' culture means it can be difficult to switch off, especially when people are firing across emails to you with requests for action. I have learned that the best response to this is to recognise what is truly urgent and what can actually wait.

Finding the right balance for you will vary depending on your personal circumstances and aspirations such as having children, starting a new career or business, or simply going through a busy work period. Achieving work-life balance doesn't mean you have to stop working hard. It is, however, about getting the balance right to create a life we love by making time as efficient as possible and knowing how and when to switch off.

When time feels restricted, it's important that we are fully aware of where our time and energy are being spent to assess what is and isn't essential. At times, we can be drawn into habits that make us less efficient and drain our energy. An example could be clicking on push notifications while trying to complete a report or spending hours scrolling through social media when you could have spent quality time with a loved one. Make an effort to check in on your digital wellbeing by setting time limits on apps that are consuming more time than you wish. Try changing your settings to only show notifications during an allocated time period or when your phone is unlocked. Alternatively, turn them off completely and check in at a set time each day using the Pomodoro technique.

If you're easily drawn into activities that are not serving you as you wish, such as certain social events or constantly supporting the needs of others before your own, then learn to say no. This can be difficult, but when you do give your time, you're likely to feel more positive and be more productive. Outsourcing the things that you're not good at or you don't enjoy doesn't just need to apply in the workplace. Housework, gardening and meal preparation are just a few tasks that can be delegated or outsourced. Remember, your version of work-life balance is likely to look different to your colleagues or your best friend, so stop comparing and find out what it is that you're striving for to excel in both your personal and professional life.

CASE STUDY: CHARLOTTE

When growing her business, Charlotte became so consumed with making it work that she says it felt like being on a never-ending treadmill that she couldn't get off. She put extreme pressure on herself to show her colleagues and staff members how hard she worked, hoping to inspire them to do the same. While it was evident that she worked incredibly hard as a business owner, this mindset placed additional pressure on her.

The feeling of being on a treadmill led to Charlotte recognising that she was heading for burnout. Since those early days of experiencing burnout, Charlotte can now identify the tell-tale signs and symptoms. She felt emotionally drained and anxious, was suffering from adrenal fatigue and was even feeling exhausted when starting the working week on a Monday morning. She developed coping mechanisms and techniques, including having a thorough checklist to help create a routine.

If you can relate to Charlotte's story, then perhaps you've found yourself feeling guilty for taking time to rest and worrying that you're not being productive enough. Try to reframe this concept and treat your rest time as you would a vacation, with no distractions from work and no agenda. Keep in the forefront of your mind that this time is for you to recharge. This will ultimately impact on your business in a positive way as you return to work fully recharged and ready to seize the day.

TASK: Finding a work-life balance

If you're interested in making a change to your current work-life balance, then work through these three questions to define a goal to help you achieve this:

- How would you feel if you were able to create the work-life balance that you desire?
- What would this look like?
- What do you need to do to achieve this?

Now define your goal.

Once you've defined what a healthy work-life balance means to you, it's important to set clear boundaries. Stick to your schedule of priorities as discussed in Chapter 7, with plotted time for work and leisure activities.

Switching off

At the end of a busy day, finding time to relax is essential in preparation for a good night's sleep. Often easier said than done, having the ability to 'switch off' from the day's activities can allow your mind to rest and rejuvenate, as well as helping to achieve a work-life balance.

When you get home from work, change your mindset to 'switch off' mode. This could involve changing to more relaxing clothes, doing some exercise, cooking a healthy meal, taking a relaxing bath or having story time with the kids. As you wind down and prepare for sleep, consider which activities help you to feel relaxed, as well as potential bad habits that could be preventing you from fully winding down.

Studies have shown that within five minutes of switching the lights off for bed, 37% of adults check their phones, rising to 60% of under thirty-fives.[47] By managing your digital wellbeing, you can make best use of digital technology while also knowing when it's time to disconnect. As part of your bedtime routine, plan when you will stop looking at your phone. This can also help prevent exposure to the bright light of a phone screen which has been recognised to stimulate the part of the brain that is designed to keep you awake. Using a clock as an alarm rather than your phone is another technique to help prevent you from looking at your phone during the night and first thing in the morning.

FOLLOW-UP WITH SOPHIE

Like many entrepreneurs, 'switching off' is something Sophie struggles with, but she does have some advice. 'I do read before bed every night without exception, which helps me to switch off. I also prioritise sleep, which gives me lots of energy for the next day. When I feel like I am becoming overwhelmed, I book a holiday or take time out. I also enjoy lots of spa days. I have a solid circle of business mates who get it and provide support when needed.'

Overthinking

Learning how to switch off can take some practice, especially if you tend to overthink. You may feel that continually thinking about something that is troubling you will lead to finding the best solution, but what usually happens is that the longer you think about the problem, the more exhausting it becomes. Recognise if you're imagining the worst-case scenario or second-guessing yourself. Neither are helpful behaviours. Other reasons for overthinking include worrying about future events such as a work deadlines and things out of your control such as a global pandemic. Signs of overthinking include being unable to relax, feeling constantly worried or anxious, experiencing negative thoughts, fixating on a particular thought and imagining worst-case scenarios. Not only do repetitive thoughts interfere with the clarity you may be seeking, but the more you worry and ruminate, the stronger a habit it becomes. If you find yourself overthinking try the following:

- **Recognise it:** Start by recognising the thought as simply a thought. Thoughts don't always speak the truth. They don't have to overwhelm you, or make you feel stressed or anxious.

- **Challenge:** Are your thoughts backed up by facts or do they have a negative or exaggerated spin?

- **Write it down or talk about it:** Writing down your thoughts can sometimes help to get them out of your head and help you to relax. If you'd like to become more self-aware of your thoughts then try keeping a log to recognise them, build self-confidence, practise self-acceptance and address any issues of concern. Sometimes, talking things through with a supportive friend is just what you need to offload, see things from a new perspective and feel more positive.

Getting into a routine of switching off can help you to relax and feel a greater sense of balance.

Self-care

Self-care is an important task that you should perform regularly to help maintain good health and wellbeing, but leading a busy lifestyle can often mean that implementing self-care becomes the last priority. When you have numerous responsibilities and an ever-growing to-do list, spending time on yourself may feel self-indulgent. However, making time to participate in activities that nurture your health and wellbeing will be far more beneficial than neglecting this area of your life.

Self-care involves taking a moment to check in with your body, feel if things are out of alignment and then implement enjoyable activities that will support your health and wellbeing. Because self-care looks different to everyone, it's important to find activities that are effective for you. Consider what activities will help 'recharge your batteries' and help you to operate at your optimal level. Plan time for self-care into your weekly schedule. It might be ten minutes before you go to bed each night or an hour on a Sunday afternoon. Find a time that works for you and aim to stick to it. Listed below are just a few self-care activity ideas. Try a couple that stand out for you:

- **Journalling:** The process of journalling can enhance your ability to cope with intrusive or avoidant thoughts through reflection. This can help to organise your thoughts, providing greater clarity and meaning. A 2018 study found that adults who journal for fifteen minutes, three times a week for twelve weeks were less likely to ruminate and were better able to move past anxious thoughts.[48] Using gratitude in your journal is another way to reap the benefits of this process, including increased happiness, stronger relationships and improved sleep.

- **Treat yourself to a massage:** Introducing massage into your routine can help with relaxation and improve overall health. Studies have shown that massage can help boost circulation in the body, alongside reducing blood pressure and boosting the immune system.[49] If you'd like to introduce regular massage into your routine but find it difficult to schedule frequent visits to a massage therapist, then why not try self-massage techniques. A foam roller is great for massaging the legs and lower back and a simple tennis ball can work wonders on the shoulders and back. There are also a wide variety of specially designed self-massage tools available to purchase.

- **Listen to music:** Through music we experience a range of emotions, such as joy, calmness or even sadness. Listening to your favourite music can help your body to relax. Try creating a playlist that you can use specifically for winding down after a busy day.

- **Meditate:** Meditation can help relax the body and the mind for a harmonised state of calm. Our brains can often become overworked in our daily routines, so the use of meditation techniques is a great way of calming down after a busy day.

- **Meet new people:** Being sociable can help improve confidence levels and self-esteem, while also encouraging communicational skills that are important in both the workplace and at home. Perhaps attend a class or activity that you otherwise might not have considered.

- **Go for a walk:** As discussed in Chapter 6, participating in exercise is really good for us. It supports improved sleep quality, increased fitness levels, and reduced stress, protects against anxiety and can improve self-esteem. Walking is one form of exercise that most of us can fit into our daily routine. Joining a walking group is a good way to stay motivated, while also making great social connections. Consider going for a walk on your next lunch break. Perhaps ask a colleague or friends to join and also start reaping the benefits.

FOLLOW-UP WITH CHARLOTTE

Each morning Charlotte uses just five minutes of her time to practise three minutes of exercise and one minute for meditation. She says, 'I try to do all of these things first thing in the morning within five minutes – otherwise they don't happen!' Keeping this time commitment short ensures consistency, so even on the busiest of days Charlotte has managed to keep this routine going.

'This way guarantees thirty-five minutes a week no matter what, and if I have time for more, I can do it,' she says. Charlotte then blocks out time where she can for other self-care activities, including walks in nature with her children, reading, listening to podcasts and taking a muscle-relaxing bath.

Summary

Balancing that equilibrium of a healthy working life can be difficult, but if you know the tricks to assist you, you'll never go back to all work and no play. Consider the following statements:

- Understand what work-life balance means to you. Know when to put the laptop down, to stop reading texts and emails and to turn the social media notifications off.

- Notice when your mind is working overtime and challenge any negative or intrusive thoughts.

- Finally, learn to switch off from the day's activities by testing some of the techniques detailed in this chapter and see what works best for you.

NINE
Reward

Having something to look forward to increases your motivation and makes it easier to follow through with even the most challenging of tasks. **Rewarding** yourself is a great way to release positive emotions and adopt healthy behaviours. This section of the PROSPER model will help you explore intrinsic and extrinsic motivation concepts, along with ways to apply them to the Stages of Change model.

Implementing behaviour change

Whether you're looking to implement a new fitness regime, regularly practise mindfulness or reduce procrastination, understanding your behaviour and the factors that might influence it can help you to develop an effective intervention strategy. When looking to make a change, finding where to start can be overwhelming and result in no action being taken at all. Sometimes, we know what we need to do and why we need to do it, but making a large change can be difficult. It requires the ultimate goal to be broken down into smaller parts and requires careful planning and ongoing commitment. Research demonstrates that even small, long-term behaviour changes can lead to significant improvements in an individual's health and life expectancy.[50]

The transtheoretical model

Behaviour change requires you to alter your behaviour until it becomes a habit. The Transtheoretical model (also known as the stages of change) was developed in the late 1970s by Prochaska and DiClemente.[51] The model outlines six stages of behaviour change and is widely used by health professionals and coaches today to provide required targeted intervention at each stage. Individuals who successfully move through the first five stages of the transtheoretical model are more likely to reach their goals and adopt positive habits. Moving from one stage to the next can take months at a time, so patience and perseverance is key. Using the transtheoretical model steps below, try and identify what stage you're at to begin any changes you would like to make for a healthier lifestyle:

1. **Pre-contemplation:** At this stage, the individual has no desire to change their behaviour. This could be due to a lack of confidence in their ability, potentially as a result of previous failed attempts or lack of understanding. They may also be unaware of the consequences of their current behaviour. An example of this is an individual needing to exercise more regularly for health reasons, but feeling overwhelmed as to where to start. They're concerned about their ability to exercise without injuring themselves and can't yet fully see the benefits physical activity could have on their health and wellbeing. If you're in this stage, then a shift in

perspective is required to move on to the contemplation stage.

2. **Contemplation:** At the contemplation stage, an individual can see the benefits of changing their behaviour and intends to do so in the next six months. They are also aware of the challenges they may face, which can ultimately prevent them from moving on to the preparation stage. An example of this is an individual who has been told by their doctor that they need to do regular exercise and has been made aware of the importance of this on their health and wellbeing. Although the individual can see that the pros outweigh the cons, they still struggle to take the first steps. If you're in this stage, then it's important to identify the things that could be holding you back and develop a strategy when you're ready to make a change.

3. **Preparation:** As an individual moves into the preparation stage, they have usually taken steps to prepare for change, such as enquiring about an exercise class, purchasing a self-help book or joining a support network. The individual is taking small, positive steps and planning to

make a change to their behaviour within the next month. If you're in this stage, it's important to analyse what challenges you may come up against so that you can develop an effective strategy to overcome them. Setting SMART (Specific, Measurable, Achievable, Relevant and Timebound) goals will also help you to stay on track.

4. **Action:** At the action stage, an individual is likely to have experienced some improvement to their health or wellbeing as a result of the ongoing changes they have made. This stage lasts around three to six months. If you're in this stage, recognise that challenges can still take you off course, so it's important to refer back to your strategy and reward yourself for your achievements.

5. **Maintenance:** As an individual enters this stage, they have maintained their behaviour change for six months. As they are now practising this behaviour regularly, they are able to maintain it with less effort than during the previous action stage. If you're in this stage, you will feel more confident about sticking to your behaviour, but accept that relapses may

happen and have a plan in place to deal with this.

6. **Relapse:** Relapse can happen at any stage and take you back to any of the previous stages in the model. It's what you do after a relapse and how you react to it that matters. Reflect on what happened when you relapsed. What were the barriers and how can you overcome these next time? Keep your vision in mind and continue to work your way through each stage of the model.

At each point that you encounter success, remember to reward yourself. Keep your goals as specific as possible. Focus on what you will gain (such as a healthier body) and how you will feel (for example, happy and energised) once you have achieved this.

Internal and external rewards

As well as rewarding yourself for reaching your milestones in achieving healthier behaviour habits, it's also important to reward yourself in your working role. Rewarding yourself is a great way to release positive emotions, adopt healthy behaviours and boost motivation. It is motivation that provides the drive to do something, so it should be ingrained into your daily routine with rewards supporting this, be they intrinsic or extrinsic.

Intrinsic motivation

Intrinsic motivation involves taking action to do something purely for the satisfaction or enjoyment that you receive. Using your internal drive, this personally rewarding task will inspire and energise you. Intrinsic motivation is important for persistence, exploring all possibilities, overcoming obstacles and seeing a task through to completion.

There are a number of ways to ensure that you're benefiting from activities that provide intrinsic reward. Start by considering what parts of your work are most meaningful for you. As a business owner, you're often pulled in multiple directions from reviewing the business finances to developing a sales strategy. The areas of your work that you're most passionate about can get lost in the mix of everything else. If you can relate to this, then become increasingly conscious of when you're carrying out tasks that are meaningful for you and, if possible, structure your day around these to enhance your feeling of purpose. Developing your knowledge or skills in this area can also provide intrinsic benefits. This could consist of enrolling on an online course, attending a weekend seminar or retreat, finding a mentor or going back into education.

As a passionate business owner, I'm sure you take pride in what you, do but how often do you take a step back and actually admire your work? Feeling pride from what you've accomplished is another way of receiving intrinsic reward and a boost to motivation.

Intrinsic motivation comes from within. In contrast, extrinsic motivation comes from external, tangible rewards. Research has shown that intrinsic motivation is generally more effective in the long term for feelings of fulfilment,[52] but both extrinsic and intrinsic motivation can differ in effectiveness based on each individual and the task at hand.

Extrinsic motivation

Extrinsic motivation is doing something for an external reward, usually financial or tangible rewards such as bonuses or a new company car. Extrinsic motivation can also include recognition and praise by others. The avoidance of punishment, for example filing a tax return to avoid a penalty, can also be considered as extrinsic motivation. They are classed as extrinsic because they originate from an outside source.

Extrinsic motivation is beneficial as it can help provide a secure income and a lifestyle you may be aspiring towards. The concept of extrinsic reward can also be helpful when you need to complete a task that doesn't motivate you intrinsically and you don't find particularly enjoyable. It's important to be mindful that extrinsic motivation can interfere with intrinsic motivation. It can lead to lower levels of persistence and creativity and even lead to burnout. The next case study is a great example of how intrinsic and extrinsic motivation can work together to achieve success.

CASE STUDY: MIKE

Mike was born and raised during the communist era of Hungary. No one had much money and his family and others didn't even have freezers in their homes. Western brands like Coca-Cola were non-existent in communist Hungary. Something changed for Mike when he saw how life could be outside a communist state. He says, 'You would see in western films, people with money and status, and it became a childhood dream.'

Mike left Hungary as a young adult with his sights set on the UK. He had no relatives or friends there and spoke little to no English. He managed to find work in a factory and shortly after, he secured a job at the pizza company, Dominos, aged twenty-one. He loved the culture of the company and the atmosphere there. He was surrounded by other young people and was motivated by the targets set by the company. Inspired by his boss, who 'drove a nice car', he could see a clear path to achieving his childhood dream.

Through hard work and climbing the ladder, Mike set up his first Dominos franchise in 2006. He now owns a range of businesses with a hundred outlets across the UK, employing more than 2,500 people and has a turnover of more than £100m. Throughout his journey, Mike says he has been able to use extrinsic reward alongside a clear mission and strong values for both his staff and himself.

Having a good mix of both intrinsic and extrinsic motivation can provide you with the support needed to achieve your goals in the short and long term. Both motivations have their place and the key is to recognise which one to use in each specific situation.

Summary

As we come to the end of the PROSPER model, the transtheoretical method (stages of change) is an approach to implement a change – something you may have identified wanting to make throughout this process.

- Using the stages of change model, identify what stage you're at and develop techniques to move on to the next stage to ultimately reach your goal.

- Reflect on intrinsic and extrinsic motivation to identify ways to reward yourself and successfully overcome obstacles that may lie ahead.

Conclusion

The PROSPER model has been your guide to working through seven key characteristics required to balance your working life with your health and wellbeing. The opportunity to reflect and take stock through a selection of reflective practices, wellbeing theories and techniques will have given you the knowledge and empowerment to structure your working day and week in the most efficient way. This will help you to reap the rewards not only for your business, but also for your health, wellbeing and relationships. No longer will 'burnout' be a barrier to your success.

We initially focused on how to prevent burn-out by learning to effectively manage stress, which can reduce your risk of long-term health issues such as heart disease, anxiety and depression. Understanding your triggers and using coping techniques that are effective for you as an individual can help you to better manage stress and ultimately avoid burnout.

Psychology is another important factor when it comes to maintaining your health and well-being and preventing burnout. We explored three theories based on positive psychology that can help you to fulfil your potential. Being comfortable in your own skin can help you to achieve a healthy mind and body.

Recognising your purpose not only provides you with a greater sense of meaning, but also helps you to maintain a good standard of health and wellbeing. By taking pleasure in what you have in life, business and relation-ships and being grateful for them through happiness and gratitude techniques, you now have the toolkits at your fingertips to enhance your positive feelings.

Having resolve is an essential attribute for an entrepreneur when avoiding burnout.

Knowing how to deal with overwhelm, procrastination and the dreaded imposter syndrome can help build a stronger 'you' when you need to focus on achieving your goals. The tools shared will assist you in maintaining a relaxed, focused and confident approach to your work, meaning dither, delay and self-doubt will no longer hold you back from realising your dreams and ambitions.

When it comes to opinion, being defined and well structured is vital as an entrepreneur. You have to be decisive and, at times, make decisions at breakneck speed. The best way to do this is to stay authentic and true to your values when casting your opinions. Focus your mind on who you are, what you are about and what you stand for. This will help you to remain authentic.

A healthy body is essential for everyday living, but it's also something that you must nurture, just like an Olympic athlete or astronaut is required to in order to achieve optimal performance. Staying physically active and getting adequate amounts of sleep can be the difference between you feeling tired and unmotivated, to feeling refreshed and raring to go. The techniques shared can help you to set yourself goals and build set times for exercising into your routine. As well as impromptu activities within the workplace or at home, incorporate the great outdoors where you can and get a good night's rest each evening.

Following the PROSPER model can be key to developing a strong, healthy mind through the application of a number of techniques. Although keeping your mind healthy can be tough, especially when you have tight deadlines, challenging encounters and lots of personalities to juggle in your business life, using techniques such as mindfulness, positivity and gratitude can provide a sense of calm and clarity when life seems hectic or overwhelming.

Productivity is key to the success of any flourishing business and the PROSPER model helps you to set the scene for that to happen. This includes considering the setup of your workspace, surrounding yourself with positive and supportive people, and also knowing when and how to deal with individuals having a negative effect on you.

Finding equilibrium in a healthy working life can be difficult, but by having tools and techniques to assist, you'll know how to make the most of your time and when to put the laptop down. Recognising when your mind is working overtime and how to challenge any negative or intrusive thoughts will help you to switch off, enjoy your downtime and come back to work feeling revitalised and raring to go.

As we come to the end of the PROSPER model, the transtheoretical model provides a tried and tested technique to implement a change. Reflecting on intrinsic and extrinsic motivation will help you to identify ways to reward yourself in achieving positive behaviour change, to motivate you in accomplishing your business goals and successfully overcoming obstacles that may lie ahead.

As you continue on your entrepreneurial journey, refer back to the PROSPER model as and when required as a supportive guide in helping you to achieve your greatest ambition without the sacrifice of your health, wellbeing or relationships. I wish you good health, success and happiness.

Notes

1 'Burn-out an "occupational phenomenon":
   International classification of diseases', WHO
   (28 May 2019), www.who.int/news/item/28-05-
   2019-burn-out-an-occupational-phenomenon-
   international-classification-of-diseases, accessed 5
   December 2022

2 Taylor-Brown, R, 'Burnout: Openview highlights
   how to keep our stress levels down', The Leaders
   Council (23 December 2021), www.leaderscouncil.
   co.uk/news/burnout-openview-highlights-
   how-to-keep-our-stress-levels-down, accessed 5
   December 2022

3 'Stress', The Mental Health Foundation (no date),
   www.mentalhealth.org.uk/explore-mental-
   health/a-z-topics/stress, accessed 5 December
   2022

4 White, JV and Gupta, VK, *Stress and Wellbeing in
   Entrepreneurship: A critical review and future research
   agenda* (Emerald Publishing Ltd, 2020)

5 Russo, MA, et al, 'The physiological effects of slow breathing in the healthy human', *Breathe*, 13/4 (2017), 298–309, https://pubmed.ncbi.nlm.nih.gov/29209423, accessed 16 December 2022

6 Fontane Pennock, S, 'Who is Martin Seligman and what does he do', PositivePsychology.com (20 September 2016), https://positivepsychology.com/who-is-martin-seligman, accessed 29 November 2022

7 Ackerman, CE, 'What is positive psychology & why is it important?', PositivePsychology.com (20 April 2018), https://positivepsychology.com/what-is-positive-psychology-definition, accessed 29 November 2022

8 Oppong, T, 'Good social relationships are the most consistent predictor of a happy life', Thrive Global (18 October 2019), https://community.thriveglobal.com/relationships-happiness-well-being-life-lessons, accessed 5 December 2022

9 Fredrickson, BL and Levenson, RW, 'Positive emotions speed recovery from the cardiovascular sequelae of negative emotions', *Cognition and Emotion*, 12/2 (1998), 191–220, https://pubmed.ncbi.nlm.nih.gov/21852890, accessed 16 December 2022

10 'Maslow's hierarchy of needs', GoodTherapy (updated 14 December 2015), www.goodtherapy.org/blog/psychpedia/maslow-hierarchy-needs, accessed 5 December 2022

11 Davis, M, '9 self-actualized historical figures', Big Think (23 July 2019), https://bigthink.com/neuropsych/9-self-actualized-historical-figures, accessed 29 November 2022

12 Rogers, C, et al, *Person to Person: The problem of being human; a new trend in psychology* (Real People Press, 1967)

13 McLeod, SA, 'Carl Rogers' humanistic theory of personality development', Simply Psychology (5 February 2014), www.simplypsychology.org/carl-rogers.html, accessed 29 November 2022

14 Rea, M and Tabor, D, 'Health state life expectancies
by national deprivation deciles, England: 2018
to 2020 census', ONS (25 April 2022), www.
ons.gov.uk/peoplepopulationandcommunity/
healthandsocialcare/healthinequalities/bulletins/
healthstatelifeexpectanciesbyindexofmultipledepri
vationimd/2018to2020, accessed 5 December 2022

15 Cherry, K, 'What is happiness? Defining
happiness, and how to become happier',
verywellmind (7 November 2022), www.
verywellmind.com/what-is-happiness-4869755,
accessed 5 November 2022

16 Kringelbach, ML and Berridge, KC, 'The
neuroscience of happiness and pleasure', *Social
Research*, 77/2 (2010), 659–678, www.ncbi.nlm.
nih.gov/pmc/articles/PMC3008658, accessed
5 December 2022

17 Newman, KM, 'How much of your happiness is
under your control?', *Greater Good Magazine*
(18 February 2020), https://greatergood.
berkeley.edu/article/item/how_much_of_your_
happiness_is_under_your_control, accessed 5
February 2022

18 Shatz, I, 'Parkinson's law: Get more done
by giving yourself less time to do things',
Effectiviology (no date), https://effectiviology.
com/parkinsons-law, accessed 5 February 2022

19 'Sleeping well', Royal College of Psychiatrists
(no date), www.rcpsych.ac.uk/mental-health/
problems-disorders/sleeping-well, accessed 5
February 2022

20 Owens, A, 'What is imposter syndrome?', Psycom
(22 December 2021), www.psycom.net/imposter-
syndrome, accessed 5 February 2022

21 Drayton, M, *The Saboteur at Work: How the
unconscious mind can sabotage ourselves, our
organisations and society* (Taylor & Francis, 2022)

22 Holt, J, 'Time bandits: What were Einstein
and Gödel talking about?', *New Yorker*

(20 February 2005), www.newyorker.com/
magazine/2005/02/28/time-bandits-2, accessed
5 February 2022

23 Young, V, 'The 5 types of impostor syndrome',
The Impostor Syndrome Institute (no date),
https://impostorsyndrome.com/articles/5-types-
of-impostors, accessed 30 November 2022

24 Brafman, R, 'Does authenticity lead to
happiness?', Psychology Today (18 August
2008), www.psychologytoday.com/gb/blog/
dont-be-swayed/200808/does-authenticity-lead-
happiness, accessed 19 December 2022

25 Solomon, RC, *Living with Nietzsche: What the great
'immoralist' has to teach us*, (Oxford University
Press, 2004)

26 Original source in German: 'Was mich nicht
umbringt, macht mich starker' (*Twilight of the
Idols*, 1888), https://libquotes.com/friedrich-
nietzsche/quote/lbw0l9e, accessed 5 February
2022

27 'Daily time spent on social networking by internet
users worldwide from 2012 to 2022', Statista
(no date), www.statista.com/statistics/433871/
daily-social-media-usage-worldwide, accessed 5
February 2022

28 Suni, E, 'How much sleep do we really need?',
Sleep Foundation (updated 29 August 2022),
www.sleepfoundation.org/how-sleep-works/
how-much-sleep-do-we-really-need, accessed
30 November 2022

29 Suni, E, 'Stages of sleep', Sleep Foundation
(updated 8 July 2022), www.sleepfoundation.org/
stages-of-sleep, accessed 5 February 2022

30 'Physical inactivity', British Heart Foundation (no
date), www.bhf.org.uk/informationsupport/risk-
factors/physical-inactivity, accessed 5 February
2022

31 'Physical activity prevents chronic disease', CDC
(2020), www.cdc.gov/chronicdisease/resources/

infographic/physical-activity.htm, accessed 5
February 2022

32 Cook, R, 'The relationship between nature and
dementia', Lifted (2 September 2021), www.
liftedcare.com/the-relationship-between-nature-
and-dementia, accessed 5 December 2022

33 Ristic, A, '15 health benefits of sunlight + dangers
& safety tips', SelfHacked (updated 14 October
2022), https://selfhacked.com/blog/avoiding-
sun-will-kill-14-proven-science-based-health-
benefits-sun, accessed 5 February 2022

34 Raman, R, 'How to safely get vitamin D from
sunlight', Healthline (28 April 2018), www.
healthline.com/nutrition/vitamin-d-from-sun,
accessed 5 February 2022

35 'Vitamin D', NHS (no date), www.nhs.uk/
conditions/vitamins-and-minerals/vitamin-d,
accessed 5 February 2022

36 Hölzel, B, et al, 'Mindfulness practice leads to
increases in regional brain grey matter density',
Psychiatry Research, 191/1 (2011), 36–43, www.ncbi.
nlm.nih.gov/pmc/articles/PMC3004979, accessed
19 December 2022

37 Emmons, RA and McCullough, ME, 'Counting
blessings versus burdens: An experimental
investigation of gratitude and subjective
well-being in daily life', *Journal of Personality
and Social Psychology*, 84/2 (2003), 377–389,
https://greatergood.berkeley.edu/pdfs/
GratitudePDFs/6Emmons-BlessingsBurdens.pdf,
accessed 5 February 2022

38 Siegle, S, 'The art of kindness', Clinic
Health System (29 May 2020), www.
mayoclinichealthsystem.org/hometown-health/
speaking-of-health/the-art-of-kindness, accessed
5 February 2022

39 Smiles, S, *Duty: With Illustrations of Courage,
Patience, and Endurance* (Harper & Brother, 1880)

40 Luenendonk, M, 'How lighting affects productivity and mood', Cleverism (25 September 2019), www.cleverism.com/how-lighting-affects-productivity-and-mood , accessed 5 February 2022

41 Chudleigh, H, 'Benefits of house plants and 7 tips for growing them', SelectHealth (no date), https://selecthealth.org/blog/2021/07/benefits-of-house-plants, accessed 5 February 2022

42 Lee, K, 'The science of single-tasking: How focus unlocks extreme productivity', Buffer (5 August 2014), https://buffer.com/resources/single-tasking, accessed 5 February 2022

43 'The Pomodoro Technique', todoist (no date), https://todoist.com/productivity-methods/pomodoro-technique, accessed 5 February 2022

44 Deane, J, 'Self-employment review: An independent report', Open Government Report (14 February 2016), www.gov.uk/government/publications/self-employment-review, accessed 5 February 2022

45 Mushtaq, R, et al, 'Relationship between loneliness, psychiatric disorders and physical health? A review on the psychological aspects of loneliness', *Journal of Clinical and Diagnostic Research*, 8/9 (2014), WE01 -WE04, https://pubmed.ncbi.nlm.nih.gov/25386507, accessed 16 December 2022

46 Jansen, M, 'The seven challenge areas for work-life balance', Life Coach Directory (6 January 2016), www.lifecoach-directory.org.uk/memberarticles/the-7-challenge-areas-for-work-life-balance, accessed 5 February 2022

47 Pearce, K, '100 mind-blowing smartphone addiction statistics', DIYGenius (5 September 2022), www.diygenius.com/smartphone-addiction-factsheet, accessed 5 December 2022

48 Smyth, JM, et al, 'Online positive affect journaling in the improvement of mental distress and well-being in general medical patients with elevated anxiety symptoms: A preliminary randomized controlled trial', *JMIR Mental Health*, 5/4 (2018), e11290, https://pubmed.ncbi.nlm.nih.gov/30530460, accessed 16 December 2022

49 'Interesting facts about massage', Pure Health (no date), https://purehealth.ie/interesting-facts-about-massage, accessed 5 February 2022

50 Celestine, N, 'What is behavior change in psychology? 5 models and theories', PositivePsychology.com (14 August 2021), https://positivepsychology.com/behavior-change, accessed 5 February 2022

51 Celestine, N, 'What is behavior change in psychology? 5 models and theories', PositivePsychology.com (14 August 2021), https://positivepsychology.com/behavior-change, accessed 5 February 2022

52 Herrity, J, 'Intrinsic vs. extrinsic motivation: What's the difference?', Indeed (10 April 2019), www.indeed.com/career-advice/career-development/intrinsic-extrinsic-motivation, accessed 5 February 2022

Acknowledgements

I'd like to acknowledge and thank the following people for help and support during the writing of *Don't Burn Out, Stand Out*: Rachael Bishop, Alice Hall, Sophie Milliken, Charlotte Nichols, Mike Racz, Simone Roche MBE, Dr Bill Scott OBE and Lou Willis-Keeler.

The Author

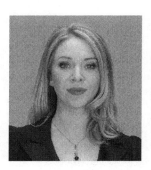

Bethany Ainsley is a corporate wellbeing specialist, coach and entrepreneur. Her journey as an entrepreneur, like many others, has been a steep learning curve. Bethany has developed an in-depth understanding of her passion and purpose, mindset and lifestyle habits that help her to be at her most productive. Together with techniques to help her relax and make the most of downtime, this has been essential in helping Bethany develop multiple businesses, alongside supporting others.

For more than a decade, Bethany and her team have provided award-winning services that have helped thousands of people improve their health and wellbeing. Their efforts were recognised in 2015 when they were awarded The David Goldman Prize for Innovation for their work in behaviour change, having helped individuals of all ages and backgrounds make healthy lifestyle choices for long-lasting results. More recently, Bethany was presented with a Director of the Year Award from the Institute of Directors for the development of their employee wellbeing software and services, supporting businesses to achieve enhanced employee wellbeing, happiness and productivity.

🌐 https://bethanyainsley.com

in https://uk.linkedin.com/in/bethanyainsley

🐦 https://twitter.com/bethanyainsley

📷 www.instagram.com/bethanyainsley/?hl=en